Transnational and Transdisciplinary Lessons of COVID 19 From the Perspective of Risk and Management

Transnational and Transdisciplinary Lessons of COVID 19 From the Perspective of Risk and Management

Editors

Julien S. Baker
Yang Gao
Alistair Cole
Emilie Tran
Xiao-Guang Yue

MDPI • Basel • Beijing • Wuhan • Barcelona • Belgrade • Manchester • Tokyo • Cluj • Tianjin

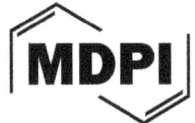

Editors

Julien S. Baker
Sport, Physical Education and Health
Hong Kong Baptist University
Kowloon Tong
Hong Kong

Yang Gao
Sport, Physical Education and Health
Hong Kong Baptist University
Kowloon Tong
Hong Kong

Alistair Cole
Government and International Studies
Hong Kong Baptist University
Kowloon Tong
Hong Kong

Emilie Tran
Government and International Studies
Hong Kong Baptist University
Kowloon Tong
Hong Kong

Xiao-Guang Yue
Professor of Computer Science
European University Cyprus
Nicosia
Cyprus

Editorial Office
MDPI
St. Alban-Anlage 66
4052 Basel, Switzerland

This is a reprint of articles from the Special Issue published online in the open access journal *Journal of Risk and Financial Management* (ISSN 1911-8074) (available at: www.mdpi.com/journal/jrfm/special_issues/COVID19_Risk).

For citation purposes, cite each article independently as indicated on the article page online and as indicated below:

LastName, A.A.; LastName, B.B.; LastName, C.C. Article Title. *Journal Name* **Year**, *Volume Number*, Page Range.

ISBN 978-3-0365-5704-5 (Hbk)
ISBN 978-3-0365-5703-8 (PDF)

© 2022 by the authors. Articles in this book are Open Access and distributed under the Creative Commons Attribution (CC BY) license, which allows users to download, copy and build upon published articles, as long as the author and publisher are properly credited, which ensures maximum dissemination and a wider impact of our publications.

The book as a whole is distributed by MDPI under the terms and conditions of the Creative Commons license CC BY-NC-ND.

Contents

About the Editors vii

Preface to "Transnational and Transdisciplinary Lessons of COVID 19 From the Perspective
of Risk and Management" ix

Alistair Cole, Julien S. Baker, Emilie Tran and Yang Gao
Introduction to the Special Issue 'Transnational and Transdisciplinary Lessons of COVID-19
from the Perspective of Risk and Management'
Reprinted from: *J. Risk Financial Manag.* 2022, 15, 210, doi:10.3390/jrfm15050210 1

**Frédéric Dutheil, Valentin Navel, Julien S. Baker, Emilie Tran, Alistair Cole and Binh Quach
et al.**
Transnational and Transdisciplinary Lessons from the COVID-19 Pandemic
Reprinted from: *J. Risk Financial Manag.* 2021, 14, 483, doi:10.3390/jrfm14100483 7

Julien S. Baker, Alistair Cole, Dan Tao, Feifei Li, Wei Liang and Jojo Jiao et al.
The Preventive Role of Exercise on the Physiological, Psychological, and Psychophysiological
Parameters of Coronavirus 2 (SARS-CoV-2): A Mini Review
Reprinted from: *J. Risk Financial Manag.* 2021, 14, 476, doi:10.3390/jrfm14100476 11

Wei Liang, Yanping Duan, Min Yang, Borui Shang, Chun Hu and Yanping Wang et al.
Behavioral and Mental Responses towards the COVID-19 Pandemic among Chinese Older
Adults: A Cross-Sectional Study
Reprinted from: *J. Risk Financial Manag.* 2021, 14, 568, doi:10.3390/jrfm14120568 23

**Frédéric Dutheil, Maelys Clinchamps, Julien S. Baker, Rashmi Supriya, Alistair Cole and
Yang Gao et al.**
Financial Burden and Shortage of Respiratory Rehabilitation for SARS-CoV-2 Survivors: The
Next Step of the Pandemic?
Reprinted from: *J. Risk Financial Manag.* 2022, 15, 20, doi:10.3390/jrfm15010020 37

Julien S. Baker, Rashmi Supriya, Dan Tao and Yang Gao
Alcohol Consumption Pre and Post COVID-19. Implications for Health, Underlying
Pathologies, Risks and Its Management
Reprinted from: *J. Risk Financial Manag.* 2021, 14, 533, doi:10.3390/jrfm14110533 43

Huw D. Wiltshire, Rashmi Supriya and Julien S. Baker
COVID-19 Impact on the Sport Sector Economy and Athletic Performance
Reprinted from: *J. Risk Financial Manag.* 2022, 15, 173, doi:10.3390/jrfm15040173 47

**Jiao Jiao, Rashmi Supriya, Bik C. Chow, Julien S. Baker, Frédéric Dutheil and Yang Gao et
al.**
COVID-19: Barriers to Physical Activity in Older Adults, a Decline in Health or Economy?
Reprinted from: *J. Risk Financial Manag.* 2022, 15, 51, doi:10.3390/jrfm15020051 53

**Hijrah Nasir, Valentin Navel, Julien S Baker, Rashmi Supriya, Alistair Cole and Yang Gao et
al.**
COVID-19: An Economic or Social Disease? Implications for Disadvantaged Populations
Reprinted from: *J. Risk Financial Manag.* 2021, 14, 587, doi:10.3390/jrfm14120587 59

Paul Chaney and Christala Sophocleous
Trust, Transparency and Welfare: Third-Sector Adult Social Care Delivery and the COVID-19 Pandemic in the UK
Reprinted from: *J. Risk Financial Manag.* **2021**, *14*, 572, doi:10.3390/jrfm14120572 . . . . **63**

Alistair Cole, Julien S. Baker and Dionysios Stivas
Trust, Transparency and Transnational Lessons from COVID-19
Reprinted from: *J. Risk Financial Manag.* **2021**, *14*, 607, doi:10.3390/jrfm14120607 . . . . **77**

Jean-Pierre Cabestan
The COVID-19 Health Crisis and Its Impact on China's International Relations
Reprinted from: *J. Risk Financial Manag.* **2022**, *15*, 123, doi:10.3390/jrfm15030123 . . . . **93**

Emilie Tran and Yu-chin Tseng
To Trust or Not to Trust? COVID-19 Facemasks in China–Europe Relations: Lessons from France and the United Kingdom
Reprinted from: *J. Risk Financial Manag.* **2022**, *15*, 187, doi:10.3390/jrfm15040187 . . . . **105**

About the Editors

Julien S. Baker

Professor Julien Steven Baker Ph.D., D.Sc. is Head of the Sport, Physical Education and Health Department at Hong Kong Baptist University. He is also the Director of the Centre for Health and Exercise Science Research. Professor Baker has published over 600 articles in peer reviewed journals. His research areas include, oxidative stress, immune function, hormonal control of exercise, metabolism, cardiovascular disease, diabetes and obesity, vascular biology, and biomechanics. He is a Fellow of the Physiological Society, and has fellowships with the Royal Society of Biology, the Human Biology Association, the Institute of Clinical Research and the Institution of Engineering and Technology. Prof Baker is also a member of the American Physiological Society, and the Society for the Study of Biology (SSOB). In addition, he has membership of the British Pharmacological Society, and the Federation of American Societies for Experimental Biology (FASEB). Professor Baker is a Honorary Professor at the University of Ningbo, and has Visiting Professor status at the University of Sydney and Ningbo University Ninth Hospital Medical Research Centre.

Prof Baker's research has attracted considerable interest from the public and media with several articles published in the Times, Scottish Herald, The Scotsman, Daily Telegraph, The Independent, The Australian, The Guardian, Daily Mail, Daily Mirror, South Wales Echo, Scottish Evening News, and Western Mail. Prof Baker had also been interviewed by BBC Radio 4, Radio 2, Radio Wales, Dragon Radio, Bristol Radio, and Scottish News.

Yang Gao

Yang GAO (Gemma) is an Associate Professor of the Department of Sport, Physical Education and Health, Hong Kong Baptist University. She is also the Director of the Centre for Health and Exercise Science Research. Dr. Gao was trained as a doctor in Preventive Medicine in the Chinese Mainland (Shandong Medical University, China) and got her Ph.D. in Medical Sciences (the Chinese University of Hong Kong, Hong Kong). Dr. Gao has been proactively involved in studies in public health and exercise sciences with diverse study designs (such as cross-sectional, case-control, cohort, RCT, systematic review, meta-analysis). In the past five years, she has obtained 15 research grants (over HK$ 5m) and published over 100 articles in international peer-reviewed journals.

Alistair Cole

Alistair Cole is Professor of Politics and Head of the Department of Government and International Studies at Hong Kong Baptist University, Before his arrival in Hong Kong in 2019, he was Professor of Politics at Cardiff University, United Kingdom (1999–2019), and Professor of Political Science at the institute of Political Studies in Lyon, France (2015–2019). He has published extensively in the field of comparative politics, public policy and area studies. Professor Cole is a graduate of Oxford University (D.Phil., 1986) and the London School of Economics (BSc econ, 1980). He is a Fellow of the Academy of Social Sciences, a Fellow of the Learned Society of Wales and a Fellow of the Royal Society of Arts. He is a frequent contributor to the media, including the BBC, Sky News, France Info, Radio France International, and RTHK.

Emilie Tran

Dr Emilie Tran is Director of Transdisciplinary Undergraduate Proggrammes, Hong Kong Baptist University (HKBU). Prior to joining HKBU in 2016, she was at the University of Saint Joseph, where she used to be the Coordinator of the Master's Programme in Government and International Studies, Head of the Department of Public Administration and International Relations, and Dean of the Faculty of Administration and Leadership. Driven by international and multidisciplinary collaborations, Dr Tran's scholarship investigates contemporary China: China's public and digital diplomacy, relations with the EU, France and the Maghrib, and transnational diaspora governance, trust and the smart city. She publishes in leading international journals, such as China Perspectives, Journal of Contemporary China, International Migration, Mediterranean Politics. She is now co-editing two handbooks with Brill Publishers, one on the overseas Chinese in Europe, and the other on the overseas Chinese in the Middle East and Africa.

Dr Tran won HKBU's highest accolade, the President's Award for Outstanding Performance in Teaching. In recognition of her 20 years of remarkable service to education, research and community service, the French Republic bestowed Dr Tran a "Knighthood"[Chevalier] of L'Ordre des Palmes Académiques, a national merit order that honours distinguished academics.

Xiao-Guang Yue

Prof. Dr. Gabriel, Xiao-Guang Yue is the Adjunct Full Professor of Computer Science at European University Cyprus and Minjiang Chair Professor of Management in China. He is an Elected Fellow of Pakistan Academy of Engineering, Foreign Member of Georgian Academy of Natural Sciences, Fellow of Royal Society of Arts. He was the Advisor to Rector, European University Cyprus, Nicosia, Cyprus. Now he is the International Advisor of CTI, Frankfurt–New York–Vienna–Bengaluru–Hong Kong. His research, spanning intelligent information processing, safety engineering and sustainability, has resulted numerous publications in refereed international journals, proceedings and book chapters. According to Scopus, he has published 122 articles, with 1100+ citations.

Preface to "Transnational and Transdisciplinary Lessons of COVID 19 From the Perspective of Risk and Management"

This reprint is the fruit of an exceptional collaboration within and beyond Hong Kong Baptist University. It is drawn from the special issue of the *Journal of Risk and Financial Management* on "Transnational and Transdisciplinary lessons from COVID-19 from the Perspective of Risk and Management". Many of the articles reproduced here were first presented as papers at the international conference organized on this theme at Hong Kong Baptist University on 20–21 May 2021. Using the related prisms of medical and social ethics, health and well-being, risk and resilience and trust and transparency panelists were invited to address questions in relation to the main lessons to be drawn from the COVID-19 crisis (in the medical, scientific, physiological, political, economic, educational, international, cultural, environmental, legal, or other domains). Experts from a broad range of academic disciplines (health, sports sciences, political science, law, geography, business, media and communication, and international relations) participated in the conference. There was, moreover, a very real international dimension to the proceedings, which is captured in this book. The transnational dimension of the symposium was reflected in the conference themes, as well by the participation of overseas speakers from the UK, France, Australia, and Singapore, as well as a range of stakeholders from outside of academia (for example, the European Union Office of Hong Kong and Macao).

The conference Transnational and Transdisciplinary Lessons from the COVID-19 Pandemic (giving rise to this Special Issue) was supported by a grant from the PROCORE-France/Hong Kong Joint Research Scheme sponsored by the Research Grants Council of Hong Kong and the Consulate General of France in Hong Kong (Reference F-HKBU205/20), as well as by the Hung Hin Shiu Charitable Foundation, by the Hong Kong Baptist University Research Committee (Project 165234), and by the Heinrich Böll Stiftung (Hong Kong). We thank these funders for their generous support. We also thank the European Union office of Hong Kong and Macao, which hosted a reception and provided speakers.

The spirit of the reprint (and the papers in the Special Issue) is to address the transdisciplinary challenges posed by the COVID-19 pandemic. Responding to existential dilemmas, the COVID-19 pandemic calls for a major transdisciplinary research effort that necessarily combines several levels of empirical analysis and methodological tools and bridges distinct academic and scientific traditions. The main sections of the reprint provide specific insights from medical and social sciences, health and well-being, politics, and society and international relations. Though the chapters are framed in terms of distinct disciplinary perspectives and traditions, the overarching spirit of the reprint to open up received wisdoms and paradigms to challenges from scholars working in different academic disciplines and traditions. The editors sincerely hope that they have met this ambition. We acknowledge all the presenters and participants of the conference "Transnational and transdisciplinary lessons of COVID-19 from the perspective of risk and management", as well as to the editorial board of the *Journal of Risk and Financial Management* in general and to Kaia LV and Scarlett Liu in particular, who expedited affairs in an efficient and courteous manner.

Julien S. Baker, Yang Gao, Alistair Cole, Emilie Tran, and Xiao-Guang Yue
Editors

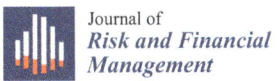

Editorial

Introduction to the Special Issue 'Transnational and Transdisciplinary Lessons of COVID-19 from the Perspective of Risk and Management'

Alistair Cole [1,*], Julien S. Baker [2], Emilie Tran [1] and Yang Gao [2]

[1] Department of Government and International Studies, Hong Kong Baptist University, Hong Kong, China; emilietran@hkbu.edu.hk

[2] Department of Sports, Physical Education and Health, Hong Kong Baptist University, Hong Kong, China; jsbaker@hkbu.edu.hk (J.S.B.); gaoyang@hkbu.edu.hk (Y.G.)

* Correspondence: alistaircole@hkbu.edu.hk

Citation: Cole, Alistair, Julien S. Baker, Emilie Tran, and Yang Gao. 2022. Introduction to the Special Issue 'Transnational and Transdisciplinary Lessons of COVID-19 from the Perspective of Risk and Management'. *Journal of Risk and Financial Management* 15: 210. https://doi.org/10.3390/jrfm15050210

Received: 8 April 2022
Accepted: 21 April 2022
Published: 5 May 2022

Publisher's Note: MDPI stays neutral with regard to jurisdictional claims in published maps and institutional affiliations.

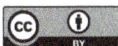

Copyright: © 2022 by the authors. Licensee MDPI, Basel, Switzerland. This article is an open access article distributed under the terms and conditions of the Creative Commons Attribution (CC BY) license (https://creativecommons.org/licenses/by/4.0/).

Rarely has scientific research been as solicited as in the past two years, as societies struggle to cope with the coronavirus. The questions raised by COVID-19 are germane to the medical and the social sciences. From an International Relations perspective, COVID-19 gets to the heart of what comprises a common good—the global commons. From a public policy perspective, COVID-19 is the wicked policy problem par excellence, requiring inter-agency collaboration. From a comparative politics perspective, COVID-19 provides a vast living dataset to engage in multi-level comparisons and real-time experiments. In the medical research field, the pandemic has provided advancements in medical science that would not have been possible without access to a living laboratory. The huge advances in medical science have themselves been filtered by societal dynamics such as trust and transparency, or risk and resilience, themes that feature in several papers in this Special Issue.

Responding to existential dilemmas, the COVID-19 pandemic calls for a major transdisciplinary research effort that necessarily combines several levels of empirical analysis and methodological tools and bridges distinct academic and scientific traditions. Such was the ambition of the conference Transnational and Transdisciplinary lessons from COVID-19, organized at Hong Kong Baptist University on 20–21 May 2021, which forms the basis for many of the articles in this Special Issue. Participants included presenters from a range of Hong Kong institutions—Hong Kong Baptist University, Hong Kong University, City University of Hong Kong, the Chinese University of Hong Kong and the Hong Kong University of Science and Technology. The international dimension of the conference was reflected in the conference themes, as well by the participation of overseas speakers from the United Kingdom (Cardiff University, Cardiff Metropolitan University, Queen Mary's, University of London); France (the Institutes of Political Studies of Paris, Aix-en-Provence and Lyon, and from the University Hospital of Clermont Ferrand); Australia (Griffith University, Monash University, Queensland University) and Singapore (National University of Singapore), as well as a range of stakeholders from outside of academia (for example, Bruegel, Water Futures Pty Ltd., European Union Office of Hong Kong and Macao). The conference organizers invited communications which addressed cutting-edge issues at the transdisciplinary and/or transnational intersection on the COVID-19 pandemic. The resulting Special Issue is focused on distinct clusters of articles, each concerned with discrete dimensions of the COVID-19 pandemic.

The first cluster of articles centers on the physiological, psychological and psychophysiological implications of COVID-19 (Baker et al. 2021a, 2021b; Dutheil et al. 2021, 2022; Liang et al. 2021; Nasir et al. 2021). In their paper, Baker et al. (2021a) refer to the cross-national evidence from lockdowns and confinements that COVID-19 has presented a serious challenge to the psychological well-being of individuals, especially in terms of their primary networks (friends, family) and practices (as a result of social distancing). Even within these tight personal networks, evidence from scholars working on psychological indicators points to an increase in indicators of social tension, such as divorce, gender violence and isolation as a result of the COVID-19 crisis. Increases in social violence and violation by communities in relation to social distancing measures are major concerns in relation to public perceptions and information provided by respective governments and their representatives. Findings converged in the sense of developing new protocols based on tele-exercise, moderate physical exercise, the selective use of Chinese medicine in a restorative capacity and focused diet.

The problem with the disease is that it effects both psychological and physiological parameters in infected populations. While the physiological parameters are easier to deal with in response to medication, psychological problems may be more of a long-term problem. This is particularly true in individuals with a history of depressive illness. Depression affects all in society, inclusive of all ages and gender. The physiological and psychological effects of COVID-19 in the long-term are currently unknown. Medical trials have been underway since the onset of the pandemic and different combinations of medication have had some beneficial effects. Drug regimens that relate to boosting the immune system and decreasing inflammation have a particular role to play. However, the treatment of depressive symptoms and illness is more complicated. There have been many medical interventions employed including pharmaceutical and medical treatments. Of course, the most successful to date has been vaccination. Interestingly, the general population's physical activity levels were recoded as low in most cases. Physical activity increases immune function, decreases symptoms associated with depressive illness and contributes to euphoria and increased well-being. Therefore, increased physical activity levels pre- and post- the pandemic may have contributed to better outcomes for patients suffering from COVID-19.

The conference keynote, on "COVID-19 and top athletic performance", was delivered by Huw Wiltshire, SFHEA, Former National Performance Director with Welsh and Russian Rugby Unions. In his speech, Dr Wiltshire stressed the importance of specific types of training for elite-level athletes—essential to avoid injury through rapidly losing fitness in the event on inactivity–or "de-training". Specific sets of issues arise for this type of actor and the COVID-19 pandemic raises more general issues about the survival of whole sports (avoiding mass contact), as well as consequences for top athletes at the individual level (Wiltshire et al. 2022).

The second cluster of articles are concerned with the related issues of trust, transparency, civil society, and governance and adopt a broad comparative perspective. Chaney and Sophocleous (2021) discuss the case of welfare trust and delivery in the four nations of the United Kingdom: England, Scotland, Wales, and Northern Ireland. The COVID-19 pandemic accelerated a number of trends in the administration of welfare policy and involvement of voluntary sector players. Each administration (the three devolved governments and the UK government operating for England) adopted a distinctive approach towards the provision of social care, undertaken by the local government tier in each respective country. Insofar as the four administrations reacted in distinctive manners, the case of COVID-19 could be considered as a natural experiment.

There are distinctive territorial ideologies in relation to welfare. In Scotland, the principle of free provision at the point of delivery is one of the binding articles of faith of Scottish devolution, and Wales follows in a broadly similar manner. In England and Northern Ireland, there is less faith in civil society or state provision, and the private sector is called upon to deliver most adult social care services, albeit under regulation from local government. In each case, there is a strong argument that COVID-19 strengthened forms of territorialization of public policy, underpinned by distinctive party systems in each of the four countries. There was a surge in volunteering action as a result of the pandemic. However, the argument prevailed in Wales and Scotland that "like-trust-like", whereby local volunteers were welcomed because it was felt they shared the same characteristics as those who needed care. A form of welfare nationalism could be observed within the

UK, setting the four nations against each other, strengthened by travel bans from entering different parts of the country.

In their paper, Cole, Baker and Stivas engage with the relationships between Trust, Transparency and Transnational lessons from COVID-19. International health crises require efforts to rebuild trust, understood in a multi-disciplinary sense as a relationship based on trusteeship in the sense of mutual obligations in a global commons, where trust is a key public good (Cole et al. 2021). The most effective responses in a pandemic are joined up ones, where individuals (responsible for following guidelines) trust intermediaries (health professionals) and are receptive to messages (nudges) from the relevant governmental authorities. Hence, the distinction between hard medical and soft social science blurs when patients and citizens are required to be active participants in combatting the virus. Building on the diagnosis of a crisis of trust (in the field of health security and across multiple layers of governance), Cole, Baker and Stivas renew with calls to restore trust by enhancing transparency.

COVID-19 raises important issues that ought to fall within the scope of international law: these include, inter alia, the lack of a common response across countries, uncertainty over vaccines and the civil responsibility of politicians in the context of a risk culture that emphasizes precaution. In fact, international health law is mainly of the soft variety. It is highly fragmented across political systems. There are competing types of law—hard and soft—but also competing standards. One conclusion of the COVID-19 pandemic might be that the crisis will push for more global norms. On the other hand, articles in this Special Issue emphasize more the zero-sum and competitive nature of international relations, far from a mutually respected and transparent legal order. Indeed, the pandemic is likely to have implications for the international power structure. Some countries, especially China, emerge relatively unaffected by the pandemic, while the majority of the other countries of the world are struggling to keep their economies running.

According to Cabestan, in his article, it is important to keep a sense of proportion. The reshuffling of the international power structure predated COVID-19 and China has been attempting to position itself as the leader of the Global South for decades in order to enhance its planetary influence (Cabestan 2022). Of course, there has been very little international cooperation over COVID-19, which has formed part of the battle of narratives between China and the West (the US in particular). However, Cabestan argues that China has engaged in "overkill". The "empire du milieu" is suspected by many of attempting to use the world Health Organization for its national interests. China's actions antagonized countries, especially as the EU, US and UK had offered substantial support to deal with the early phases of the pandemic. As captured by the Pew survey, public opinion has moved against China in most European countries, though less so elsewhere. The controversy over the vaccines also rebounded against China, as the quality of the vaccines it delivered (and that of medical material such as masks) was not up to standard. All in all, Cabestan used the example of COVID-19 to illustrate broader trends of competition between China and the West in an increasing zero-sum environment.

Tran and Tseng, in their article, continue the discussion on China's health diplomacy (Tran and Tseng 2022). Combining critical juncture theory and (dis)trust in international relations, they examine how facemasks became a politicized object, both between states and between Mainland China and its overseas population, as the epidemic unfolded throughout Europe. Their interdisciplinary and mixed-methods approach (international relations, framing analysis, semi-structured interviews, and digital ethnography) unveils how the COVID-19 outbreak impacted China–Europe relations, comparing two European settings: France and the United Kingdom. They argue that the common denominator appears to be the reduced trust, if not outright distrust, between individuals and communities in the French and British contexts, and in Sino–French and Sino–British relations at the transnational level.

A selection of the conference papers is presented in this Special Issue, along with some other cognate contributions produced by the call for papers.

The conference was organized by Hong Kong Baptist University's Department of Government and International Studies, in association with the Department of Sport, Physical Education and Health and the David C Lam Institute for East–West Studies. It was generously supported by Hung Hin Shiu Charitable Foundation; by the David C Lam Institute for East–West Studies; by the PROCORE (French Consulate of Hong Kong-Macao and Research Grants Council of Hong Kong), by the Hong Kong Baptist University Research Committee, by the European Union Office of Hong Kong and Macao and by the Heinrich Böll Stiftung Hong Kong. We are grateful to these funders, and especially to the Heinrich Böll Stiftung of Hong Kong and Macao and the Hong Kong Baptist University Research Committee, which funded the papers in this Special Issue. We offer our sincere thanks to all of these funders, as well as to the editorial board of the Journal of *Risk and Financial Management* in general and to Kaia LV and Scarlett Liu in particular, who expedited affairs in an efficient and courteous manner.

Author Contributions: A.C. mainly wrote the manuscript; J.S.B., E.T. and Y.G. contributed to discussion and editing. All authors have read and agreed to the published version of the manuscript.

Funding: The conference Transnational and Transdisciplinary Lessons from the COVID-19 Pandemic (giving rise to this special issue) was supported by a grant from the PROCORE-France/Hong Kong Joint Research Scheme sponsored by the Research Grants Council of Hong Kong and the Consulate General of France in Hong Kong (Reference F-HKBU205/20), as well as by the Hung Hin Shiu Charitable Foundation, by the Hong Kong Baptist University Research Committee (Project 165234), and by the Heinrich Böll Stiftung (Hong Kong). We thank these funders for their generous support.

Institutional Review Board Statement: Not applicable.

Informed Consent Statement: Not applicable.

Data Availability Statement: Not applicable.

Acknowledgments: We acknowledge all the presenters and participants of the conference "Transnational and transdisciplinary lessons of COVID-19 from the perspective of risk and management".

Conflicts of Interest: The authors declare no conflict of interest.

References

Baker, Julien S., Alistair Cole, Dan Tao, Feifei Li, Wei Liang, Jojo Jiao, Yang Gao, and Rashmi Supriya. 2021a. The Preventive Role of Exercise on the Physiological, Psychological, and Psychophysiological Parameters of Coronavirus 2 (SARS-CoV-2): A Mini Review. *Journal of Risk and Financial Management* 14: 476. [CrossRef]

Baker, Julien S., Rashmi Supriya, Dan Tao, and Yang Gao. 2021b. Alcohol Consumption Pre and Post COVID-19. Implications for Health, Underlying Pathologies, Risks and Its Management. *Journal of Risk and Financial Management* 14: 533. [CrossRef]

Cabestan, Jean-Pierre. 2022. The COVID-19 Health Crisis and Its Impact on China's International Relations. *Journal of Risk and Financial Management* 15: 123. [CrossRef]

Chaney, Paul, and Christala Sophocleous. 2021. Trust, Transparency and Welfare: Third-Sector Adult Social Care Delivery and the COVID-19 Pandemic in the UK. *Journal of Risk and Financial Management* 14: 572. [CrossRef]

Cole, Alistair, Julien S. Baker, and Dionysios Stivas. 2021. Trust, Transparency and Transnational Lessons from COVID-19. *Journal of Risk and Financial Management* 14: 607. [CrossRef]

Dutheil, Frédéric, Valentin Navel, Julien S. Baker, Emilie Tran, Alistair Cole, Binh Quach, Jiao Jiao, Jean-Baptiste Bouillon-Minois, and Maëlys Clinchamps. 2021. Transnational and Transdisciplinary Lessons from the COVID-19 Pandemic. *Journal of Risk and Financial Management* 14: 483. [CrossRef]

Dutheil, Frédéric, Maelys Clinchamps, Julien S. Baker, Rashmi Supriya, Alistair Cole, Yang Gao, and Valentin Navel. 2022. Financial Burden and Shortage of Respiratory Rehabilitation for SARS-CoV-2 Survivors: The Next Step of the Pandemic? *Journal of Risk and Financial Management* 15: 20. [CrossRef]

Liang, Wei, Yanping Duan, Min Yang, Borui Shang, Chun Hu, Yanping Wang, and Julien Steven Baker. 2021. Behavioral and Mental Responses towards the COVID-19 Pandemic among Chinese Older Adults: A Cross-Sectional Study. *Journal of Risk and Financial Management* 14: 568. [CrossRef]

Nasir, Hijrah, Valentin Navel, Julien S Baker, Rashmi Supriya, Alistair Cole, Yang Gao, and Frederic Dutheil. 2021. COVID-19: An Economic or Social Disease? Implications for Disadvantaged Populations. *Journal of Risk and Financial Management* 14: 587. [CrossRef]

Tran, Emilie, and Yu-chin Tseng. 2022. To Trust or not to Trust? Facemasks in China-Europe Relations, Lessons from France and the United Kingdom. *Journal of Risk and Financial Management* 15: 187. [CrossRef]

Wiltshire, Huw, Rashmi Supriya, and Julien S. Baker. 2022. COVID 19 Impact on the Sport Sector Economy and Athletic Performance. *Journal of Risk and Financial Management* 14: 173. [CrossRef]

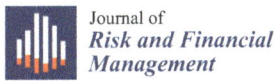

Editorial

Transnational and Transdisciplinary Lessons from the COVID-19 Pandemic

Frédéric Dutheil [1,2], Valentin Navel [3], Julien S. Baker [4], Emilie Tran [4], Alistair Cole [4], Binh Quach [4], Jiao Jiao [4], Jean-Baptiste Bouillon-Minois [5] and Maëlys Clinchamps [1,*]

1 CNRS, LaPSCo, Physiological and Psychosocial Stress, University Clermont Auvergne, Preventive and Occupational Medicine, University Hospital of Clermont-Ferrand, F-63000 Clermont-Ferrand, France; fred_dutheil@yahoo.fr
2 WittyFit, F-75000 Paris, France
3 CNRS, INSERM, GReD, University Clermont Auvergne, Ophthalmology, University Hospital of Clermont-Ferrand, F-63000 Clermont-Ferrand, France; valentin.navel@hotmail.fr
4 Centre for Health and Exercise Science Research, Physical Education and Health, Hong Kong Baptist University, Kowloon Tong, Hong Kong 999077, China; jsbaker@hkbu.edu.hk (J.S.B.); emilietran@hkbu.edu.hk (E.T.); alistaircole@hkbu.edu.hk (A.C.); bquach@hkbu.edu.hk (B.Q.); jojojiao@hkbu.edu.hk (J.J.)
5 CNRS, LaPSCo, Physiological and Psychosocial Stress, University Clermont Auvergne, Emergency Medicine, University Hospital of Clermont-Ferrand, F-63000 Clermont-Ferrand, France; jbb.bouillon@gmail.com
* Correspondence: mclinchamps@chu-clermontferrand.fr

Citation: Dutheil, Frédéric, Valentin Navel, Julien S. Baker, Emilie Tran, Alistair Cole, Binh Quach, Jiao Jiao, Jean-Baptiste Bouillon-Minois, and Maëlys Clinchamps. 2021. Transnational and Transdisciplinary Lessons from the COVID-19 Pandemic. *Journal of Risk and Financial Management* 14: 483. https://doi.org/10.3390/jrfm14100483

Received: 23 September 2021
Accepted: 7 October 2021
Published: 13 October 2021

Publisher's Note: MDPI stays neutral with regard to jurisdictional claims in published maps and institutional affiliations.

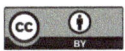

Copyright: © 2021 by the authors. Licensee MDPI, Basel, Switzerland. This article is an open access article distributed under the terms and conditions of the Creative Commons Attribution (CC BY) license (https://creativecommons.org/licenses/by/4.0/).

On 7 January 2020, China identified a virus called severe acute respiratory syndrome coronavirus 2 (SARS-CoV-2). This disease was classified as COVID-19 by the World Health Organization. WHO experts admit that the hypothesis that the coronavirus was transmitted by a first animal and then a second before contamination of humans is "most likely". Because they have played a central role in the emergence of various viral diseases (Gupta et al. 2021), bats were quickly suspected. With 1400 species of bats (20% of all species of mammals), the diversity of the species is highly favorable to the emergence of new viruses. Because they fly, share human environments and have a long-life expectancy, the idea is widespread that bats carry many viruses, but this is not sufficient to threaten humans. Proportionally, bats do not carry a higher number of zoonotic pathogens, normalized by species richness, compared with other mammalian and avian species. Objectively identified evidence that bats carry more viruses that infect humans is needed to identify the pandemic source (Dutheil et al. 2021a). To fight the increase in cases, local authorities of affected areas established quarantine periods and containment that we could compare with those of submariners (Bouillon-Minois et al. 2020a). This resulted in a decrease in industrial activities, mass transit and individual car circulation. Consecutively to these restrictions, NASA scientists have documented a reduction in pollutants firstly in China (30% NO_2, 25% CO_2) then across the world (Dutheil et al. 2020a). Therefore, the coronavirus seems to be the first disaster with benefits on levels of air pollution (Bouillon-Minois et al. 2020b). Air pollution is responsible for many deaths and increased incidences of respiratory disease. The public health benefit of the world's efforts to reduce transmission of SARS-CoV-2 may have indirect health benefits by reducing cardiovascular morbidity (Dutheil et al. 2020b) or respiratory diseases (Dutheil et al. 2020c) such as allergies (Navel et al. 2020a). On the other hand, restriction measures and containment could lead to several adverse effects. People can develop psychological illnesses with long-term post-traumatic disorder (Dutheil et al. 2021b; Croizier et al. 2020). The increasing time on screens can aggravate eye problems such as myopia (Navel et al. 2020b). The limitations of outdoor activity may have favored domestic violence (Bouillon-Minois et al. 2020c) and decreased physical activity related to teleworking (Thivel et al. 2021), provoking an increase in body mass index (Urzeala et al. 2021), increasing metabolic risk, aggravating the accumulation of fat mass, insulin resistance and metabolic syndrome in future months (Thivel et al. 2021). During this home lockdown, people have also experienced a slowing down of time and an increase in boredom and sadness experienced in lockdown situations (Droit-Volet et al. 2020). The fear due to the COVID-19 pandemic also had unexpected effects on the sales of guns, which were multiplied more than two time in the USA, matching the curve of the increase in cases of COVID-19 (Dutheil et al. 2020d, 2020e). The COVID-19 pandemic also exacerbated the inequalities in public health. For example, we saw local epidemics in more populated and disadvantaged areas, such as prisons (Dutheil et al. 2020f). Furthermore, COVID-19 also caused a paradoxical reduction of admissions in emergency departments that were not in areas of COVID-19 cases (Bouillon-Minois et al. 2021), or a massive decrease in annoyance and stress related to sound pollution and, therefore, potential increased cardiovascular disease (Dutheil et al. 2020g). The global worldwide lockdown was followed by a prolonged period of social distancing aiming to reduce transmission of SARS-CoV2. We observed an interesting debate on the effects of smoking on the transmission of SARS-Cov2, cigarettes being a possible support of transmission (Dutheil et al. 2020h). Finally, COVID-19 caused long-term effects (Dutheil et al. 2020). After a massive decrease in pollution, the lifting of restrictions lead to an economic growth boost. We fear that countries worldwide will choose to protect the economy rather than the environment (Dutheil et al. 2020i). Transnational and transdisciplinary lessons from the COVID-19 pandemic are yet to be made. The COVISTRESS study started before the pandemic and prior to lockdowns, and is still ongoing (Urzeala et al. 2021; Droit-Volet et al. 2020; Ugbolue et al. 2020). The COVISTRESS study aims to encompass all sectors and aspects of our lives and may promote long-term comprehension of the effects of the pandemic, and therefore contribute to effective preventive strategies.

Conflicts of Interest: The authors declare no conflict of interest.

References

Bouillon-Minois, Jean-Baptiste, Marion Trousselard, and Frédéric Dutheil. 2020a. COVID-19 pandemic containment: Following the example of military submariners. *BMJ Military Health* 166: 362. [CrossRef]
Bouillon-Minois, Jean-Baptiste, François-Xavier Lesage, Jeannot Schmidt, and Frédéric Dutheil. 2020b. Coronavirus and Exceptional Health Situations: The First Disaster With Benefits on Air Pollution. *Disaster Medicine and Public Health Preparedness* 14: e28–e30. [CrossRef]
Bouillon-Minois, Jean-Baptiste, Maëlys Clinchamps, and Frédéric Dutheil. 2020c. Coronavirus and Quarantine: Catalysts of Domestic Violence. *Violence against Women*, 1–3. [CrossRef]
Bouillon-Minois, Jean-Baptiste, Jeannot Schmidt, and Frédéric Dutheil. 2021. SARS-CoV-2 pandemic and emergency medicine: The worst is yet to come. *The American Journal of Emergency Medicine* 42: 246–47. [CrossRef]
Croizier, Caroline, Jean-Baptiste Bouillon-Minois, Jacques-Olivier Bay, and Frédéric Dutheil. 2020. COVID-19 lockdown and mental health: Why we must look into oncology units. *Psychological Medicine*, 1–2. [CrossRef] [PubMed]
Droit-Volet, Sylvie, Sandrine Gil, Natalia Martinelli, Nicolas Andant, Maëlys Clinchamps, Lénise Parreira, Karine Rouffiac, Michael Dambrun, Pascal Huguet, Benoît Dubuis, and et al. 2020. Time and Covid-19 stress in the lockdown situation: Time free, «Dying» of boredom and sadness. *PLoS ONE* 15: e0236465. [CrossRef] [PubMed]
Dutheil, Frédéric, Yolande Esquirol, and Valentin Navel. 2020. Will the COVID-19 pandemic decrease the FatMax? *Journal of Applied Physiology* 129: 1. [CrossRef] [PubMed]
Dutheil, Frédéric, Julien S. Baker, and Valentin Navel. 2020a. COVID-19 as a factor influencing air pollution? *Environmental Pollution* 263: 114466. [CrossRef] [PubMed]
Dutheil, Frédéric, Marion Trousselard, and Valentin Navel. 2020b. SARS-CoV-2 as a protective factor for cardiovascular mortality? *Atherosclerosis* 304: 64–65. [CrossRef]
Dutheil, Frédéric, Valentin Navel, and Maëlys Clinchamps. 2020c. The Indirect Benefit on Respiratory Health From the World's Effort to Reduce Transmission of SARS-CoV-2. *Chest* 158: 467–68. [CrossRef]
Dutheil, Frédéric, Julien S. Baker, and Valentin Navel. 2020d. To fight SARS-CoV-2: Putting your guns down. *Canadian Journal of Public Health* 111: 411–12. [CrossRef]
Dutheil, Frédéric, Julien S. Baker, and Valentin Navel. 2020e. Firearms or SARS-Cov-2: What is the most lethal? *Public Health* 183: 44–45. [CrossRef]
Dutheil, Frédéric, Jean-Baptiste Bouillon-Minois, and Maëlys Clinchamps. 2020f. COVID-19: A prison-breaker? *Canadian Journal of Public Health* 111: 480–81. [CrossRef]

Dutheil, Frédéric, Julien S. Baker, and Valentin Navel. 2020g. COVID-19 and cardiovascular risk: Flying toward a silent world? *Journal of Clinical Hypertension* 22: 1945–46. [CrossRef]

Dutheil, Frédéric, H. Nasir, and Valentin Navel. 2020h. SARS-CoV-2 Tackles the Tobacco Industry: Comment on "Tobacco Industry Interference Index: Implementation of the World Health Organization's Framework Convention on Tobacco Control Article 5.3 in India". *Asia Pacific Journal of Public Health* 32: 371–72. [CrossRef] [PubMed]

Dutheil, Frédéric, Julien S. Baker, and Valentin Navel. 2020i. COVID-19 and air pollution: The worst is yet to come. *Environmental Science and Pollution Research* 27: 44647–49. [CrossRef]

Dutheil, Frédéric, Maëlys Clinchamps, and Jean-Baptiste Bouillon-Minois. 2021a. Bats, Pathogens, and Species Richness. *Pathogens* 10: 98. [CrossRef] [PubMed]

Dutheil, Frédéric, Laurie Mondillon, and Valentin Navel. 2021b. PTSD as the second tsunami of the SARS-Cov-2 pandemic. *Psychological Medicine* 51: 1773–74. [CrossRef]

Gupta, Parakriti, Mini P. Singh, Kapil Goyal, Pande Tripti, Mohd Ikram Ansari, Vinodhkumar Obli Rajendran, Kuldeep Dhama, and Yashpal Singh Malik. 2021. Bats and viruses: A death-defying friendship. *Virusdisease* 32: 1–13. [CrossRef]

Navel, Valentin, F. Chiambaretta, and Frédéric Dutheil. 2020a. Will environmental impacts of social distancing due to the pandemic caused by SARS-CoV-2 decrease allergic disease? *Journal of Allergy and Clinical Immunology* 146: 70–71. [CrossRef] [PubMed]

Navel, Valentin, Steven Beze, and Frédéric Dutheil. 2020b. COVID-19, sweat, tears . . . and myopia? *Clinical and Experimental Optometry* 103: 555. [CrossRef] [PubMed]

Thivel, David, Michéle Tardieu, Pauline Genin, Alicia Fillon, Benjamin Larras, Pierre Melsens, Julien Bois, Frédéric Dutheil, Francois Carré, Gregory Ninot, and et al. 2021. COVID-19-Related National Re-confinement: Recommendations From the National French Observatory for Physical Activity and Sedentary Behaviors (ONAPS). *Journal of Physical Activity and Health* 18: 474–76. [CrossRef]

Ugbolue, Ukadike Chris, Martine Duclos, Constanta Urzeala, Mickael Berthon, Keri Kulik, Aura Bota, David Thivel, Reza Bagheri, Yaodong Gu, Julien S. Baker, and et al. 2020. An Assessment of the Novel COVISTRESS Questionnaire: COVID-19 Impact on Physical Activity, Sedentary Action and Psychological Emotion. *Journal of Clinical Medicine* 9: 3352. [CrossRef] [PubMed]

Urzeala, Constanta, Martine Duclos, Ukadike Chris Ugbolue, Aura Bota, Mickael Berthon, Keri Kulik, David Thivel, Reza Bagheri, Yaodong Gu, Julien S Baker, and et al. 2021. COVID-19 lockdown consequences on body mass index and perceived fragility related to physical activity: A worldwide cohort study. *Health Expectations*. [CrossRef]

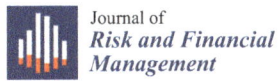

Review

The Preventive Role of Exercise on the Physiological, Psychological, and Psychophysiological Parameters of Coronavirus 2 (SARS-CoV-2): A Mini Review

Julien S. Baker [1], Alistair Cole [2], Dan Tao [1], Feifei Li [1], Wei Liang [1], Jojo Jiao [1], Yang Gao [1] and Rashmi Supriya [1,*]

[1] Centre for Health and Exercise Science Research, Department of Sport, Physical Education and Health, Hong Kong Baptist University, Kowloon Tong 999077, Hong Kong; jsbaker@hkbu.edu.hk (J.S.B.); emma0514@hkbu.edu.hk (D.T.); lifeifei@hkbu.edu.hk (F.L.); wliang1020@hkbu.edu.hk (W.L.); jojojiao@hkbu.edu.hk (J.J.); gaoyang@hkbu.edu.hk (Y.G.)

[2] Department of Government and International Studies, Hong Kong Baptist University, Kowloon Tong 999077, Hong Kong; alistaircole@hkbu.edu.hk

* Correspondence: rashmisupriya@hkbu.edu.hk

Abstract: The world has been severely challenged by the Coronavirus Disease (COVID-19) outbreak since the early 2020s. Worldwide, there have been more than 66 million cases of infection and over 3,880,450 deaths caused by this highly contagious disease. All sections of the population including those who are affected, those who are not affected and those who have recovered from this disease, are suffering physiologically, psychologically or psychophysiologically. In this paper we briefly discuss the consequences of COVID-19 on physiological, psychological and psychophysiological vulnerability. We also attempt to provide evidence in support of exercise management as a prevention strategy for improving and minimizing the physiological, psychological and psychophysiological effects of COVID-19. Moderate exercise including walking, yoga and tai-chi to name but a few exercise regimes are critical in preventing COVID-19 and its complications. Governments, public health authorities and the general population should maintain physical activity during the COVID-19 pandemic to prevent additional physical and mental distress.

Keywords: COVID-19; coronavirus disease; physiological effects; psychological effects; psychophysiological effects; exercise; physical activity

1. Introduction

There has been a global pandemic of COVID-19 since 2019. The WHO reported 3,880,450 deaths associated with COVID-19 as of 23 June 2021 (World Health Organisation 2021). COVID-19 and associated public health measures may negatively affect individuals with physical, behavioral health (mental illness, substance abuse), financial insecurity and socioeconomic vulnerability. Recent studies suggest that the measures taken to curb the spread of the COVID-19 outbreak have generated issues throughout the population (Clemente-Suárez et al. 2020; Adhikari et al. 2020). It has been established and identified that the possible risk factors are related to physiological, psychological and psychophysiological vulnerability. Research suggests that impaired immunity may be the root cause of physiological, psychological and psychophysiological vulnerability. For instance, physiological complications due to the pandemic have been reported to be severe in immune-compromised people including the obese, overweight, elderly or subjects with metabolic syndrome or underlying pathologies. Similarly, anxiety and depression, the two major psychological complications reported during the COVID-19 pandemic are influenced by inflammatory pathways and neurotransmitters that are activated by an imbalance of the immune system. Furthermore, psychophysiological vulnerability during COVID-19 including a wide variety of health disorders, such as headaches, essential hypertension, insomnia, asthma, gastrointestinal and dermatological conditions have been linked with modulation of cortisol levels and increases in pro-inflammatory cytokines. The purpose of this paper is to briefly discuss the consequences of COVID-19 on physiological, psychological and psychophysiological vulnerability; and to briefly outline the mechanisms of how exercise can help in modulating these factors. We have also attempted to provide evidence in support of exercise management as a prevention strategy for improving and minimizing the physiological, psychological and psychophysiological effects of COVID-19 (Figure 1).

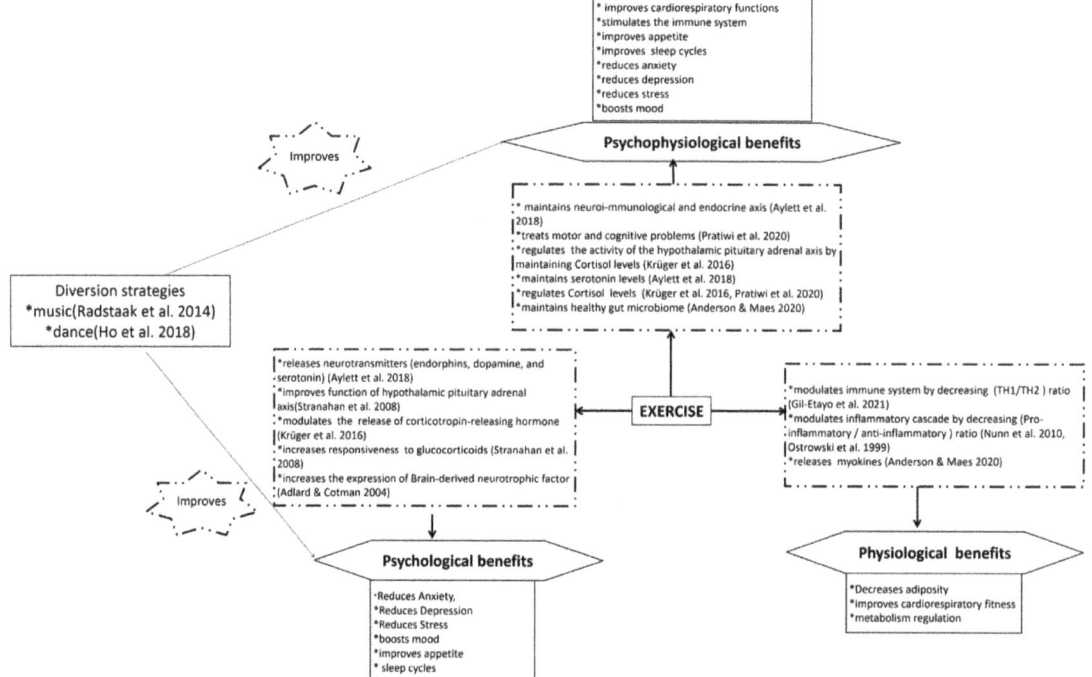

Figure 1. Summary figure showing the preventive role of exercise on physiological, psychological and psychophysiological effects of COVID-19.

2. Search Strategy

This paper was prepared from the presentation on idea presented in the symposium "Transnational and Transdisciplinary Lessons of COVID-19 From the Perspective of Risk and Management". A structured search strategy was conducted in PubMed and Google scholar to search for publications in English using the search term "COVID-19 OR SARS-CoV-2 OR CORONA" in combination with one of the following keywords: "physiological effects", "psychological effects", "psychophysiological effects", "exercise", "Yoga" and "tai chi". We focused on clinical trials, meta-analyses and review articles. We did not include research related with athletes and psychosocial factors. The search was completed on 21 June 2021. When many similar articles were available, the most recent articles were used. Additional papers were identified from random searches and the reference lists of retrieved articles. No date restriction was put on the search so that a longitudinal 'map' of the subject area could be obtained

3. Physiological Effects of COVID-19 and Its Management by Exercise

Physiological Effects of COVID-19: The pandemic has caused physiological complications mostly in elderly populations including (age $\geq$ 60 years) the obese and overweight people with body mass indexes (BMI) over 25 kg/m^2 or even higher, these individuals contribute to increased risk of infection scores for COVID-19. According to our previous review we have demonstrated that more than 50% of the population with obesity and/or overweight were admitted for critical care and had high mortality (Wang et al. 2020). The condition of obesity refers to excess body fat, low-grade chronic inflammation and impaired immunity that is associated with many debilitating and life-threatening diseases. The list includes respiratory dysfunction, cardiovascular disease, diabetes, some cancers, metabolic risk and co-morbidities, some of which have been linked to more severe COVID-19 infections (Stefan et al. 2020). Additionally, inactivity has now been identified as one of the biggest COVID-19 risk factors. Researchers studied 48,440 adults (a cross-section of the racially diverse Southern California population with an average age of 47 years) between 1 January and 21 October 2020 who were tested positive for COVID-19. The data showed that 6.4 percent of participants were consistently active while 14.4 percent were consistently inactive. Surprisingly, 79.2 percent of respondents were inconsistent exercisers. Study results found that a person who is consistently inactive has higher risk levels for COVID-19 complications. Their risk is comparable to that of people over the age of 60 and those who have undergone organ transplantation. Hospitalization rates for inactive people were twice as high as those for consistently active people. Additionally, these individuals have a 1.73 times greater chance of needing care in the intensive care unit (ICU) and a 2.49 times greater chance of dying from COVID-19 (Narici et al. 2021). Narrowing down to the molecular level, Angiotensin-converting enzyme 2(ACE2) has been identified as a receptor for COVID-19 entry. ACE2 appears to be a receptor for COVID-19, and obesity may increase ACE2 expression in lung epithelial cells. Clearly, the more adipocytes present, the more ACE2 receptors there are to spread the virus. Additionally, COVID-19 exhibits hyperactive inflammatory responses. The immune system produces pro-inflammatory cytokines Interleukins (IL-6, IL-1β, IL-2, IL-15, IL-10, IL-13) and tumor necrosis factor-alpha (TNF-alpha) in response to an infection. When a virus attacks the immune system, it damages the parenchyma of the lungs and the bronchi and triggers respiratory discomfort resulting in adverse respiratory disorders. Further, it becomes serious enough to require medication (Jose and Manuel 2020; Stebbing et al. 2020; Gil-Etayo et al. 2021). Research also suggests that increased levels of IL-15 and a high T-helper 2 response are associated with a fatal outcome related to COVID-19 (Gil-Etayo et al. 2021). Research has established a significant reduction of %T helper 1 cells and %T helper 17 cells with higher activated %T helper 2 cells in COVID-19 patients compared with controls. Senescent T helper 2 cell percentage was observed to be an independent risk factor for death (Gil-Etayo et al. 2021).

Exercise Benefits related to the Physiological Effects of COVID-19: As per our previous review we established that there are multiple advantages of exercise in relation to human health (Wang et al. 2020). These include decreased adipose tissue, improved cardio-respiratory fitness (CRF) and enhancement of metabolic homeostasis and even suppression of inflammation. The most effective way to lose weight is to increase daily energy expenditure through exercise or physical activity. Exercise, in particular, accelerates the breakdown of glycogen in the muscles and the liver; this results in the breakdown of fat in adipose tissue and muscle; and facilitates the oxidation of fatty acids in the muscles (Poirier and Després 2001). A higher CRF corresponds to a lower accumulation of visceral adipose tissue (overweight and obesity) (Brock et al. 2011). In addition, exercise improves oxygen delivery and uptake in exercising muscles. In studies involving subjects with a low baseline CRF, exercise interventions using different modalities (aerobic and resistance) at moderate intensities significantly improved CRF in overweight, obese middle-aged women and men (Church et al. 2010). In contrast, during physical inactivity, metabolic homeostasis is disrupted, leading to insulin resistance, reduced lipid clearance post-prandially, muscle decline and an increase in visceral adiposity (Pedersen and Febbraio 2012). Moreover, chronic systemic inflammation resulting from metabolic disruption has been linked to persistent physical inactivity (Nunn et al. 2010). Hence, increased exercise would help prevent metabolic derangements. It has been found that moderate-intensity exercise of at least 150 min per week can lower the prevalence of metabolic syndrome (Donnelly et al. 2009). Additionally, it has been observed in previous studies that inflammation and exercise have a negative relationship. Infection leads to the overproduction of pro-inflammatory cytokines such as interleukins (IL-6, IL-2, IL15 etc.) and TNF-alpha (Ostrowski et al. 1999). On the other hand, individuals who perform more frequent and intense physical activity have lower levels of inflammatory biomarkers (IL-6, IL-1β, and TNF-alpha). Through its unique cytokine and hormonal effects, exercise intensity may affect T helper 1/T helper 2 cell balance. Exercises such as walking, tai chi and restorative yoga stimulate the T helper 1 response (Shimizu et al. 2008; Nieman et al. 2005; Raghavendra et al. 2009; Esch et al. 2007), while more intense workouts and longer durations stimulate T helper 2. Cortisol is lowered by low-intensity exercise and relaxing activities, while it is raised by high-intensity exercise and long-duration workouts. There has been evidence that cortisol increases the development of T helper 2 cells and decreases that of T helper 1. Exercise may also push the body toward a more T helper 2 dominated state (as muscle-derived IL-6 behaves differently from TNF-alpha-associated IL-6) and associated IL-10. Muscle-derived IL-6 and associated IL-10 are anti-inflammatory (Narici et al. 2021) and enhances the body's immune response. However, low- to medium-intensity high-volume resistive exercise, that is easily implemented at home, will have positive effects, particularly if combined with a 15–25% reduction in daily energy intake. The combination of these regimens seems ideal for preserving neuromuscular, metabolic, and cardiovascular health (Narici et al. 2021). Furthermore, individuals have been advised to perform 150 min of moderate intensity exercise per week initially to obtain the necessary amount of exercise. This exercise intensity seems favorable in modifying the effects of COVID-19. A larger amount of exercise should be followed for significant weight loss and to prevent weight gain. Generally, 11,000 steps per day with 64–170 steps/minute and at least 10 min duration is sufficient for healthy adults (Wang et al. 2020).

4. Psychological Effects of COVID-19 and Its Management by Exercise

Psychological Effects of COVID-19: A state of psychological distress is a state of emotional suffering caused by stressors and demands that people have difficulty in coping with. It is usually characterized by feelings of depression and anxiety (Arvidsdotter et al. 2016). Globally, adolescents of varying backgrounds experience higher levels of anxiety, depression, and stress due to the pandemic and have become frequent consumers of alcohol and recreational drugs (Jones et al. 2021). Based on US Census Bureau, around 56.2% of adults (age = 18–24 years), 48.9% of adults (age = 25–49 years), 39.1 % adults (age = 50–66 years) and 29.3% of adults (age = 65+ years) have been reported to have anxiety and/or depressive symptoms during the pandemic (Anon 2020). The most common psychological effects of COVID-19 on the general population are depression and anxiety. Among the general population, changing social dynamics, such as social distancing, restricted movement and lockdown, have led to severe behavioral and psychological changes. Due to the imposition of lockdown, people work from home, attend online classes and are restricted from visiting established social networks, such as religious meetings, which result in people suffering from stress problems and non-regulation of emotions, that help individuals develop resilience. In addition to social changes, people also experience severe mental and emotional changes due to their fear of getting the disease and uncertainty about their futures. This results from having been confined, abnormally reduced social/physical contact with others, and losing familiar habits are all directly related to feeling distressed, bored, socially isolated and frustrated (Reynolds et al. 2008; Hawryluck et al. 2004). Frustration and loneliness can be attributed to inhibitions from daily activities, interruption of social necessities, and not participating in social network activities (Jeong et al. 2016). The prevalence of loneliness may be associated with depression and suicidal behavior

(Serafini et al. 2020). An evaluation of depression and anxiety in Hong Kong during the COVID-19 pandemic revealed that 19% of the 500 respondents had depression and 14% had anxiety. Additionally, 25.4% reported that their mental health had deteriorated since the pandemic (Choi et al. 2020). Even people who are infected with the disease mainly suffer from anxiety and depression. A study conducted in Hubei on COVID-19 patients (n = 460) revealed that 304 people were diagnosed with somatization symptoms (66.09%), followed by depression (53.48%), anxiety (46.30%), insomnia (42.01%) and self-mutilating or suicidal thoughts (23.26%) (Wang et al. 2021). Existing studies have shown that those who have been exposed to the risk of infection may develop pervasive fears about their health, worries about infecting others, and fear of infecting family members. Cognitive, emotional, and behavioral disorders are reported to be associated with gender-based differences during the COVID-19 pandemic in many studies. Mostly women showed significant higher anxiety, depression, precautionary behavior and emotional responses and acute stress levels than men (Levkovich and Shinan-Altman 2021; García-Fernández et al. 2021; Hou et al. 2020). Focusing on the molecular level, research suggests that cortisol levels were significantly higher in patients with COVID-19 than in individuals who had not contracted the disease. They suggest that COVID-19 patients with highly elevated cortisol levels are more likely to quickly deteriorate in relation to health status. Patients with a cortisol baseline level of 744 or less survived on average for 36 days. Survival was only 15 days for patients with levels over 744 (Tan et al. 2020).

Exercise Benefits on the Psychological Effects of COVID-19: Numerous studies have shown the positive effects of exercise on anxiety and depression (Ströhle 2009; Stonerock et al. 2015; Stubbs et al. 2017), and exercise is widely accepted as a non-invasive means of treating or preventing those conditions (Rosa Rimes et al. 2015; Mikkelsen et al. 2017). Relaxation techniques and breathing exercises have been recommended as an intervention for COVID-19 patients to reduce acute anxiety, although more evidence is needed (Khawam et al. 2020). It was found that aerobic exercise was effective in treating anxiety and depression in a study of exercise treatment for clinical anxiety. Exercise programs with a high intensity gain more benefits than programs with a low intensity y (Aylett et al. 2018). Some of the most helpful exercises in reducing anxiety include running, swimming, cycling, walking, dancing and even gardening (Hu et al. 2020). Exercise releases neurotransmitters in the body called endorphins, dopamine, and serotonin. They are natural chemicals produced in the brain that helps our body cope with stress. This boosts mood by releasing serotonin, improves appetite and sleep cycles (Aylett et al. 2018). The dysfunction of hypothalamic–pituitary–adrenal (HPA) axis, the increased secretion of corticotropin-releasing hormone (CRH), the impaired responsiveness to glucocorticoids, the increased size and activity of the pituitary were all observed in patients with depression. The ability of exercise on regulating HPA supported physical exercise as one of the methods to improve depressive symptoms (Stranahan et al. 2008). In contrast a study suggests that moderate-to-vigorous physical activities were negatively related to the symptoms of depression. The study proposed that increased light activity and reduced sedentary behavior might contribute to the decreased prevalence of depression (Kandola et al. 2020). At the molecular level, decreased brain-derived neurotrophic factor (BDNF) level is a vulnerability factor for anxiety (Janke et al. 2015). Numerous studies have found that physical exercise can increase the expression of BDNF in the dentate gyrus (area of the brain where all sensory parts come together to create unique representations and memories and is critical for memory and learning) (Adlard and Cotman 2004). Physical exercise was found to be able to restore BDNF to pre-stress levels, suggesting that exercise protects against stress-induced decreased levels of BDNF (Adlard and Cotman 2004). Exercise can also control inflammation, which is a possible mechanism to help reduce anxiety. As reported in a previous study, elevated levels of the pro-inflammatory cytokine C-reactive protein was associated with anxiety disorders (Vogelzangs et al. 2013). Intriguingly, exercise conferred its beneficial effect on anxiety by regulating inflammatory systems (Flynn et al. 2007). Yoga, an ancient eastern practice consisting of breath control, physical postures and meditation, has demonstrated beneficial effects in patients with severe anxiety symptoms, although the effect was relatively mild (Saeed et al. 2019). A study examined the effect of Tai Chi, a traditional Chinese martial art, on anxiety in older adults and found that those receiving medical therapy could benefit from Tai Chi exercise, but those only receiving medical therapy in isolation, could not (Song et al. 2014). As far as mental health is concerned, aerobic exercise interventions have proven to successfully to reduce depression in patients with low to moderate symptoms (Morres et al. 2019; Schuch et al. 2016). The alleviating effects of aerobic exercise interventions on self-reported depressive symptoms in clinical depression have been shown to be comparable to those of antidepressant treatments (Dinas et al. 2011; Blumenthal et al. 2007). Therefore, during the current pandemic, aerobic exercise can help to protect from an increase in depressive symptomatology in people with a diagnosis of clinical depression who already suffer from mild to moderate depressive symptoms. Exercise can also help in preventing depressive symptoms in people at risk for depression. Moreover, aerobic exercise interventions have been found to be effective in anxiety disorders (Generalized Anxiety Disorder, Panic Disorder, Obsessive-Compulsive Disorder, Social Phobia) (Aylett et al. 2018), and stress-related disorders such as post-traumatic stress disorder (Franklin and McCullough 2009), i.e., disorders that are expected to increase during the current pandemic. This psychological issue may not only occur in COVID survivors or health workers, but also the general population (Bohlken et al. 2020; Petzold et al. 2020). As far as clinical anxiety symptoms are concerned, aerobic exercise interventions do not achieve the same effects as psychopharmaceutic treatment in clinical anxiety patients (Carek et al. 2011), but it has proven itself as an adjunctive therapeutic treatment for anxiety disorders in several randomized controlled trial studies (Jayakody et al. 2014). In addition, as a means of primary prevention with respect to the current pandemic, already an acute bout of aerobic exercise of moderate intensity (>21 min) can successfully reduce anxiety (Rebar et al. 2015). Additionally, there is a mood-regulatory effect possible after just seven minutes of aerobic exercise (low to moderate intensity).

5. Psychophysiological Effects of COVID-19 and Its Management by Exercise

Psychophysiological Effects of COVID-19: Psychophysiology studies investigate the physiological effects of the psychological processes and behavior, as well as the impact of behavioral or psychological manipulations on the body. Psychophysiological measures include techniques designed to assess activity in a variety of bodily systems. As a result of psychological and psychosocial stressors/triggers, a person may experience depression, anxiety, panic attacks, somatic symptoms or posttraumatic stress disorder symptoms, delirium, psychosis or even suicidality. The term psychophysiology has been used to refer to a wide variety of disorders, such as headaches, essential hypertension, insomnia, asthma and gastrointestinal and dermatological conditions (Clemente-Suárez et al. 2020). Constrictions and restrictions mean a sudden end to citizens' normal lives. As a result, the individual begins to display symptoms of anxiety caused by social isolation, lack of mental hygiene habits and repeated exposure to negative news and information. Feelings of sadness, apathy, fear, uncertainty, frustration, irregular circadian cycles, insomnia, hyper vigilance and difficulty concentrating may accompany this illness. COVID symptomatology can trigger feelings of shame, social stigma and even guilt. The subject can mistake some symptoms, such as headaches, migraines or irritation in the throat, for COVID symptoms despite not being infected. The social isolation measures imposed by governments around the world led to a sharp decline in physical activity as recreation facilities, athletic centers, gyms, public parks, playgrounds and schools were forced to close. Furthermore, the gut microbiome may play a crucial role, since it is known that gut bacteria are responsible for mental disorders such as depression and anxiety (strongly present during the pandemic) (Anderson and Maes 2020; Keely et al. 2012). The gut microbiome may modulate the pathophysiology of COVID-19 by altering the immune system and triggering reactions (Anderson and Maes 2020). Additionally, many of the conditions that appear to increase the risk of COVID-19 fatalities are associated with altered gut permeability and dysbiosis, such as obesity, diabetes, cardiovascular disorders and lung and respiratory airway inflammation (Anderson and Maes 2020). Stress makes the population more vulnerable to viral infection by affecting the second brain, the gut microbiome (Narici et al. 2021). COVID-19 is predominantly a pulmonary condition, highlighting the importance of the gut, since previous studies have identified a gut-lung axis which suggests that respiratory infections are associated with changes in gut microbiota (Keely et al. 2012). In this way, microbial metabolites and certain endotoxins may have an impact on the lung through the bloodstream, and inflammation may have a reciprocal impact on the gut microbiota (Dumas et al. 2018). The increase in pro-inflammatory cytokines directly leads to a down regulation of hormones that maintain circadian rhythms (Markus et al. 2018). Narrowing to the molecular level there have been recent studies suggesting how psychological stress may also lead to higher levels of corticotropin-releasing hormone (CRH) in the brain, thereby contributing to cortisol production (Vanuytsel et al. 2014). CRH influences inflammatory cytokines and the production of TNF alpha, so its role in the emergence of COVID-19, and therefore its severity and fatalities, is likely to be linked to CRH. This raises the intriguing possibility that COVID-19 could also influence the gut microbiota.

Exercise Benefits on the Psychophysiological Effects of COVID-19: Exercise is not only likely to reduce stress, it also improves sleep as well, and it is a well-established fact that exercise has many benefits for overall health. General and mental health benefits of physical activity and regular aerobic exercise with respect to the functioning of the central nervous system, the peripheral autonomous nervous system, the immune system, mental health, stress and well-being have already been explored (Rosa Rimes et al. 2015). Regular aerobic exercise at a moderate level reduces respiratory tract infections because it stimulates the immune system (hormonal effects and cellular effects) (Krüger et al. 2016). Active lifestyles and regular aerobic exercise can save lives by preventing mental and physical health problems. Regarding the current SARS-CoV-2-Coronavirus pandemic, it is important to note that particularly aerobic exercise focused on endurance and cardiorespiratory fitness has positive effects on physical and mental health, particularly sports that involve large amounts of muscle. Besides stimulating the immune system (neuroimmunology and endocrine axis), it also improves cardiorespiratory functions, relieves anxiety and depression, and functions as a buffer against chronic stress by facilitating bodily recovery and reducing perceived stress symptoms. Mental and physical health are interdependent, as are physical activity's effects on both. The benefits of aerobic exercise have been observed in longitudinal and quasi-experimental studies on clinical patient groups (with neurological, somatic and mental disorders) and in healthy subjects without a history of chronic disease (Blair 1996; Franklin and McCullough 2009; Gerber and Pühse 2009; Haskell et al. 2007). During a pandemic lockdown, it is imperative for people with or without a history of lifestyle-related diseases or mental disorders to exercise regularly and stay physically active in order to avoid long-term harm to their physical and mental health. Fitness benefits are typically curvilinear and occur even with relatively low volumes of exercise. Furthermore, exercise positively impacts cognitive, daily, psychosocial and neuroendocrine functions. For instance, Tai-chi is beneficial for treating cognitive problems. Researchers have observed increased and reduced activity of the HPA axis in schizophrenia patients, though studies have shown both hyperfunction and hypofunction of the HPA axis which controls cortisol levels. They found that reducing salivary cortisol levels (a neuroendocrine indicator of stress and immunity, which can provide insights into the possible physiological mechanisms behind this effect) (Ho et al. 2014). Another study involved examining the physiological and psychological impacts of walking in urban parks throughout winter, spring, and early summer. A total of 12 middle-aged and older adults were involved in walking (11–15 min) in an urban park in Japan. To determine physiological responses, their heart rate and blood pressure were measured. The results show that walking in urban parks leads to physiological, psychological relaxation and varied landscape appreciation (Pratiwi et al. 2020). Exercise guidelines generally recommend that 150 min per week of moderate-intensity aerobic activity, such as brisk walking, and/or 75 min of vigorous-intensity exercise, such as jogging, cycling, swimming, or aerobics. A combination of resistance training, strength-endurance training and yoga, targeting large muscle groups such as the legs or the entire body, is also highly recommended.

As stress is characterized by high levels of arousal and negative effects, mood regulation is a core function of stress recovery. Therefore, mood-regulating strategy involves redirecting cognitions and actions away from the stressor, the so-called diversion strategy. Music as a diversion strategy and results in psychophysiological recovery from stress. Music has been shown to lower anxiety and improve mood. There is some evidence that different music styles can impact psychophysiological recovery differently. Compared with listening to heavy metal, listening to classical music and music selected by the listener, helps in reducing stress. It decreases anxiety and increases relaxation. Listening to classical music after a stressful event decreased systolic blood pressure (Radstaak et al. 2014). Dance movement therapy (DMT) and physical exercise were examined in a study conducted for older adults with dementia. DMT participants showed significant reductions in depression, loneliness, and negative mood, as well as improving daily functioning and the diurnal cortisol slope. At 1-year follow-up, the effects on daily functioning and the cortisol slope remained unchanged. The study results suggest that DMT can be utilized as a multifaceted intervention to improve various aspects of functioning in older adults with declining cognitive abilities (Ho et al. 2018).

The use of artificial intelligence (AI) has increased in COVID-19 research, especially in Detection, classification, severity, and mortality risk assessment. Tracking coronavirus by using AI has already demonstrated its potential to stratify high-risk patients. This technique has also proven to be effective in predicting the infection rate in real time (Rogers 2021; Phillips 2021). Physical education (PE) can also be improved by incorporating AI. A practical understanding of education based on a technical understanding educational and research activities are taking place in all fields in order to consider new ideas pertinent to their respective fields. In case of physical education technology the new ideas are lacking in comparison to other academic fields (Lee and Lee 2021). Additionally, it is crucial to build an integrated research workforce and establish an effective research infrastructure. Similarly, in order to facilitate the comprehensive advancement in exercise, we must develop an environment for modern technology development in the field of physical education, and develop overall AI-related exercise applications.

6. Conclusions

Exercise has multiple benefits in combatting the vicious cycle of the physiological, psychological and psychophysiological impacts of COVID-19. Exercise could provide stimulation for the human constitution and could provide potential benefits on resisting the virus. These measures if implemented sooner may reduce underlying pathologies and contribute to the reduction of mortality associated with the COVID-19 pandemic. The health benefits of exercise, as well as its potential to save lives, should be promoted to future generations, governments, and policymakers. Additionally, future focus should be drawn on developing an environment for AI-related exercise applications. In addition, some important considerations should be considered. It is essential to realize the importance of mind relaxation techniques using music, dance and breathing exercises in conjunction with increases in physical activity. In addition, individuals should strictly follow social distancing and avoid mass gatherings in public areas while performing exercises during the COVID-19 pandemic.

Author Contributions: J.S.B. and R.S. wrote the manuscript; J.S.B. designed the study; A.C. and D.T. F.L., J.J., W.L. and Y.G. contributed to discussion and editing. All authors have read and agreed to the published version of the manuscript.

Funding: This research received no external funding.

Institutional Review Board Statement: Not applicable.

Informed Consent Statement: Not applicable.

Data Availability Statement: Not applicable.

Acknowledgments: We acknowledge all the presenters and participants at the conference "Translational and transdisciplinary lessons of COVID-19 from the perspective of risk and management".

Conflicts of Interest: The authors declare no conflict of interest.

References

Adhikari, Sasmita Poudel, Sha Meng, Yu-Ju Wu, Yu-Ping Mao, Rui-Xue Ye, Qing-Zhi Wang, Chang Sun, Rozelle Scott, Hein Raat, Huan Zhou, and et al. 2020. Epidemiology, causes, clinical manifestation and diagnosis, prevention and control of coronavirus disease (COVID-19) during the early outbreak period: A scoping review. *Infectious Diseases of Poverty* 9: 29. [CrossRef]

Adlard, P. A., and C. W. Cotman. 2004. Voluntary exercise protects against stress-induced decreases in brain-derived neurotrophic factor protein expression. *Neuroscience* 124: 985–92. [CrossRef]

Anderson, George, and Michael Maes. 2020. Gut Dysbiosis Dysregulates Central and Systemic Homeostasis via Suboptimal Mitochondrial Function: Assessment, Treatment and Classification Implications. *Current Topics in Medicinal Chemistry* 20: 524–39. [CrossRef]

Anon. 2020. US Census Bureau, Household Pulse Survey. Available online: https://www.kff.org/coronavirus-covid-19/issue-brief/the-implications-of-covid-19-for-mental-health-and-substance-use/ (accessed on 3 September 2021).

Arvidsdotter, Tina, Bertil Marklund, Sven Kylén, Charles Taft, and Inger Ekman. 2016. Understanding persons with psychological distress in primary health care. *Scandinavian Journal of Caring Sciences* 30: 687–94. [CrossRef]

Aylett, Elizabeth, Nicola Small, and Peter Bower. 2018. Exercise in the treatment of clinical anxiety in general practice–a systematic review and meta-analysis. *BMC Health Services Research* 18: 559. [CrossRef] [PubMed]

Blair, Steven N. 1996. Influences of Cardiorespiratory Fitness and Other Precursors on Cardiovascular Disease and All-Cause Mortality in Men and Women. *JAMA Journal of the American Medical Association* 276: 205. [CrossRef] [PubMed]

Blumenthal, James A., Michael A. Babyak, P. Murali Doraiswamy, Lana Watkins, Benson M. Hoffman, Krista A. Barbour, Steve Herman, W. E. Craighead, A. L. Brosse, R. Waugh, and et al. 2007. Exercise and Pharmacotherapy in the Treatment of Major Depressive Disorder. *Psychosomatic Medicine* 69: 587–96. [CrossRef] [PubMed]

Bohlken, Jens, Friederike Schömig, Matthias R. Lemke, Matthias Pumberger, and Steffi G. Riedel-Heller. 2020. COVID-19-Pandemie: Belastungen des medizinischen Personals. *Psychiatrische Praxis* 47: 190–97. [CrossRef]

Brock, David W., Brian A. Irving, Barbara Gower, and Gary R. Hunter. 2011. Differences emerge in visceral adipose tissue accumulation after selection for innate cardiovascular fitness. *International Journal of Obesity* 35: 309–12. [CrossRef]

Carek, Peter J., Sarah E. Laibstain, and Stephen M. Carek. 2011. Exercise for the Treatment of Depression and Anxiety. *The International Journal of Psychiatry in Medicine* 41: 15–28. [CrossRef]

Choi, Edmond Pui Hang, Bryant Pui Hung Hui, and Eric Yuk Fai Wan. 2020. Depression and Anxiety in Hong Kong during COVID-19. *International Journal of Environmental Research and Public Health* 17: 3740. [CrossRef] [PubMed]

Church, Timothy S., Conrad P. Earnest, Angela M. Thompson, Elisa Priest, Ruben Q. Rodarte, Travis Sanders, Robert Ross, and Steven N. Blair. 2010. Exercise without Weight Loss Does Not Reduce C-Reactive Protein. *Medicine and Science in Sports and Exercise* 42: 708–16. [CrossRef] [PubMed]

Clemente-Suárez, Vicente Javier, Athanasios A. Dalamitros, Ana Isabel Beltran-Velasco, Juan Mielgo-Ayuso, and Jose Francisco Tornero-Aguilera. 2020. Social and Psychophysiological Consequences of the COVID-19 Pandemic: An Extensive Literature Review. *Frontiers in Psychology* 11: 3077. [CrossRef] [PubMed]

Dinas, P. C., Y. Koutedakis, and A. D. Flouris. 2011. Effects of exercise and physical activity on depression. *Irish journal of Medical Science* 180: 319–25. [CrossRef] [PubMed]

Donnelly, Joseph E., Steven N. Blair, John M. Jakicic, Melinda M. Manore, Janet W. Rankin, and Bryan K. Smith. 2009. Appropriate Physical Activity Intervention Strategies for Weight Loss and Prevention of Weight Regain for Adults. *Medicine and Science in Sports and Exercise* 41: 459–71. [CrossRef] [PubMed]

Dumas, Alexia, Lucie Bernard, Yannick Poquet, Geanncarlo Lugo-Villarino, and Olivier Neyrolles. 2018. The role of the lung microbiota and the gut-lung axis in respiratory infectious diseases. *Cellular Microbiology* 20: e12966. [CrossRef] [PubMed]

Esch, Tobias, Jorg Duckstein, Justus Welke, and Vittoria Braun. 2007. Mind/body techniques for physiological and psychological stress reduction: Stress management via Tai Chi training—A pilot study. *Medical Science Monitor* 13: CR488–CR497.

Flynn, Michael G., Brian K. McFarlin, and Melissa M. Markofski. 2007. State of the Art Reviews: The Anti-Inflammatory Actions of Exercise Training. *American Journal of Lifestyle Medicine* 1: 220–35. [CrossRef]

Franklin, Barry A., and Peter A. McCullough. 2009. Cardiorespiratory Fitness: An Independent and Additive Marker of Risk Stratification and Health Outcomes. *Mayo Clinic Proceedings* 84: 776–79. [CrossRef]

García-Fernández, Lorena, Verónica Romero-Ferreiro, Sergio Padilla, Pedro David López-Roldán, María Monzó-García, and Roberto Rodriguez-Jimenez. 2021. Gender differences in emotional response to the COVID-19 outbreak in Spain. *Brain Behavior* 11: e01934. [CrossRef]

Gerber, Markus, and Uwe Pühse. 2009. Review Article: Do exercise and fitness protect against stress-induced health complaints? A review of the literature. *Scandinavian Journal Public Health* 37: 801–19. [CrossRef]

Gil-Etayo, Francisco Javier, Patricia Suàrez-Fernández, Oscar Cabrera-Marante, Daniel Arroyo, Sara Garcinuño, Laura Naranjo, and Daniel E. Pleguezuelo. 2021. T-Helper Cell Subset Response Is a Determining Factor in COVID-19 Progression. *Frontiers in Cellular and Infection Microbiology* 11: 79. [CrossRef]

Haskell, William L., I-Min Lee, Russell R. Pate, Kenneth E. Powell, Steven N. Blair, Barry A. Franklin, Caroline A. Macera, Gregory W. Heath, Paul D. Thompson, and Adrian Bauman. 2007. Physical Activity and Public Health. *Medicine and Science in Sports and Exercise* 39: 1423–34. [CrossRef] [PubMed]

Hawryluck, Laura, Wayne L. Gold, Susan Robinson, Stephen Pogorski, Sandro Galea, and Rima Styra. 2004. SARS Control and Psychological Effects of Quarantine, Toronto, Canada. *Emerging Infectious Diseases* 10: 1206–12. [CrossRef]

Ho, Rainbow Tin Hung, Adrian Ho Yin Wan, Friendly So Wah Au-Yeung, Phyllis Hau Yan Lo, Pantha Joey Chung Yue Siu, Cathy Pui Ki Wong, Winnie Yuen Han Ng, Irene Kit Man Cheung, Siu Man Ng, Cecilia Lai Wan Chan, and et al. 2014. The psychophysiological effects of Tai-chi and exercise in residential Schizophrenic patients: A 3-arm randomized controlled trial. *BMC Complementary and Alternative Medicine* 14: 364. [CrossRef] [PubMed]

Ho, Rainbow Tin Hung, Ted C. T. Fong, Wai Chi Chan, Joseph S. K. Kwan, Patrick K. C. Chiu, Joshua C. Y. Yau, and Linda C. W. Lam. 2018. Psychophysiological Effects of Dance Movement Therapy and Physical Exercise on Older Adults With Mild Dementia: A Randomized Controlled Trial. *The Journals of Gerontology: Series B*. [CrossRef] [PubMed]

Hou, Fengsu, Fengying Bi, Rong Jiao, Dan Luo, and Kangxing Song. 2020. Gender differences of depression and anxiety among social media users during the COVID-19 outbreak in China:a cross-sectional study. *BMC Public Health* 20: 1648. [CrossRef] [PubMed]

Hu, Shaojuan, Lorelei Tucker, Chongyun Wu, and Luodan Yang. 2020. Beneficial Effects of Exercise on Depression and Anxiety During the COVID-19 Pandemic: A Narrative Review. *Frontiers in Psychiatry* 11: 1217. [CrossRef]

Janke, Kellie L., Tara P. Cominski, Eldo V. Kuzhikandathil, Richard J. Servatius, and Kevin C. H. Pang. 2015. Investigating the Role of Hippocampal BDNF in Anxiety Vulnerability Using Classical Eyeblink Conditioning. *Frontiers in Psychiatry* 6. [CrossRef]

Jayakody, Kaushadh, Shalmini Gunadasa, and Christian Hosker. 2014. Exercise for anxiety disorders: Systematic review. *British Journal of Sports Medicine* 48: 187–96. [CrossRef]

Jeong, Hyunsuk, Hyeon Woo Yim, Yeong-Jun Song, Moran Ki, Jung-Ah Min, Juhee Cho, and Jeong-Ho Chae. 2016. Mental health status of people isolated due to Middle East Respiratory Syndrome. *Epidemiology and Health* 38: e2016048. [CrossRef]

Jones, Elizabeth A. K., Amal K. Mitra, and Azad R. Bhuiyan. 2021. Impact of COVID-19 on Mental Health in Adolescents: A Systematic Review. *International Journal of Environmental Research and Public Health* 18: 2470. [CrossRef]

Jose, Ricardo J., and Ari Manuel. 2020. COVID-19 cytokine storm: The interplay between inflammation and coagulation. *The Lancet Respiratory Medicine* 8: e46–e47. [CrossRef]

Kandola, Aaron, Gemma Lewis, David P. J. Osborn, Brendon Stubbs, and Joseph F. Hayes. 2020. Depressive symptoms and objectively measured physical activity and sedentary behaviour throughout adolescence: A prospective cohort study. *The Lancet Psychiatry* 7: 262–71. [CrossRef]

Keely, Simon, Nicholas J. Talley, and Philip M. Hansbro. 2012. Pulmonary-intestinal cross-talk in mucosal inflammatory disease. *Mucosal Immunology* 5: 7–18. [CrossRef] [PubMed]

Khawam, Elias, Hassan Khouli, and Leo Pozuelo. 2020. Treating acute anxiety in patients with COVID-19. *Cleveland Clinic Journal of Medicine*. [CrossRef] [PubMed]

Krüger, Karsten, Frank-Christoph Mooren, and Christian Pilat. 2016. The Immunomodulatory Effects of Physical Activity. *Current Pharmaceutical Design* 22: 3730–48. [CrossRef] [PubMed]

Lee, Hyun Suk, and Junga Lee. 2021. Applying Artificial Intelligence in Physical Education and Future Perspectives. *Sustainability* 13: 351. [CrossRef]

Levkovich, Inbar, and Shiri Shinan-Altman. 2021. The impact of gender on emotional reactions, perceived susceptibility and perceived knowledge about COVID-19 among the Israeli public. *International Health*. [CrossRef] [PubMed]

Markus, Regina P., Pedro A. Fernandes, Gabriela S. Kinker, Sanseray da Silveira Cruz-Machado, and Marina Marçola. 2018. Immune-pineal axis—Acute inflammatory responses coordinate melatonin synthesis by pinealocytes and phagocytes. *British Journal of Pharmacology* 175: 3239–50. [CrossRef]

Mikkelsen, K., L. Stojanovska, M. Polenakovic, M. Bosevski, and V. Apostolopoulos. 2017. Exercise and mental health. *Maturitas* 106: 48–56. [CrossRef] [PubMed]

Morres, Ioannis D., Antonis Hatzigeorgiadis, Afroditi Stathi, Nikos Comoutos, Chantal Arpin-Cribbie, Charalampos Krommidas, and Yannis Theodorakis. 2019. Aerobic exercise for adult patients with major depressive disorder in mental health services: A systematic review and meta-analysis. *Depression Anxiety* 36: 39–53. [CrossRef] [PubMed]

Narici, Marco, Giuseppe De Vito, Martino Franchi, Antonio Paoli, Tatiana Moro, Giuseppe Marcolin, Bruno Grassi, Lucrezia Zuccarelli, Biolo Gianni, Filippo Giorgio Di Girolamo, and et al. 2021. Impact of sedentarism due to the COVID-19 home confinement on neuromuscular, cardiovascular and metabolic health: Physiological and pathophysiological implications and recommendations for physical and nutritional countermeasures. *European Journal of Sport Science* 21: 614–35. [CrossRef]

Nieman, David C., Dru A. Henson, Melanie D. Austin, and Victor A. Brown. 2005. Immune Response to a 30-Minute Walk. *Medicine and Science in Sports and Exercise* 37: 57–62. [CrossRef] [PubMed]

Nunn, Alistair V., Geoffrey W. Guy, James S. Brodie, and Jimmy D. Bell. 2010. Inflammatory modulation of exercise salience: Using hormesis to return to a healthy lifestyle. *Nutrition & Metabolism* 7: 87. [CrossRef]

Ostrowski, Kenneth, Thomas Rohde, Sven Asp, Peter Schjerling, and Bente Klarlund Pedersen. 1999. Pro- and anti-inflammatory cytokine balance in strenuous exercise in humans. *The Journal of physiology* 515: 287–91. [CrossRef] [PubMed]

Pedersen, Bente K., and Mark A. Febbraio. 2012. Muscles, exercise and obesity: Skeletal muscle as a secretory organ. *Nature Reviews Endocrinology* 8: 457–65. [CrossRef] [PubMed]

Petzold, Moritz Bruno, Jens Plag, and Andreas Ströhle. 2020. Umgang mit psychischer Belastung bei Gesundheitsfachkräften im Rahmen der COVID-19-Pandemie. *Nervenarzt* 91: 417–21. [CrossRef]

Phillips, Ashley. 2021. Artificial Intelligence-enabled Healthcare Delivery and Digital Epidemiological Surveillance in the Remote Treatment of Patients during the COVID-19 Pandemic. *American Journal of Medical Research* 8: 30. [CrossRef]

Poirier, Paul, and Jean-Pierre Després. 2001. Exercise In Weight Management of Obesity. *Cardiology Clinics* 19: 459–70. [CrossRef]

Pratiwi, Prita Indah, Qiongying Xiang, and Katsunori Furuya. 2020. Physiological and Psychological Effects of Walking in Urban Parks and Its Imagery in Different Seasons in Middle-Aged and Older Adults: Evidence from Matsudo City, Japan. *Sustainability* 12: 4003. [CrossRef]

Radstaak, Mirjam, Sabine A. E. Geurts, Jos F. Brosschot, and Michiel A. J. Kompier. 2014. Music and Psychophysiological Recovery from Stress. *Psychosomatic Medicine* 76: 529–37. [CrossRef] [PubMed]

Raghavendra, Rao M., H. S. Vadiraja, Raghuram Nagarathna, H. R. Nagendra, M. Rekha, N. Vanitha, and K. S. Gopinath. 2009. Effects of a Yoga Program on Cortisol Rhythm and Mood States in Early Breast Cancer Patients Undergoing Adjuvant Radiotherapy: A Randomized Controlled Trial. *Integrative Cancer Therapies* 8: 37–46. [CrossRef] [PubMed]

Rebar, Amanda L., Robert Stanton, David Geard, Camille Short, Mitch J. Duncan, and Corneel Vandelanotte. 2015. A meta-meta-analysis of the effect of physical activity on depression and anxiety in non-clinical adult populations. *Health Psychology Review* 9: 366–78. [CrossRef] [PubMed]

Reynolds, Diane L., J. R. Garay, S. L. Deamond, Maura K. Moran, W. Gold, and R. Styra. 2008. Understanding, compliance and psychological impact of the SARS quarantine experience. *Epidemiology & Infection* 136: 997–1007. [CrossRef]

Rogers, Rob. 2021. Internet of Things-based Smart Healthcare Systems, Wireless Connected Devices, and Body Sensor Networks in COVID-19 Remote Patient Monitoring. *American Journal of Medical Research* 8: 71. [CrossRef]

Rosa Rimes, Ridson, Marcos de Souza Moura Antonio, Murilo Khede Lamego, Alberto Souza de Sa Filho, Joao Manochio, Flavia Paes, and Mauro Giovanni Carta. 2015. Effects of Exercise on Physical and Mental Health, and Cognitive and Brain Functions in Schizophrenia: Clinical and Experimental Evidence. *CNS Neurological Disorders-Drug Targets (Formerly Current Drug Targets-CNS & Neurological Disorders)* 14: 1244–54. [CrossRef]

Saeed, Sy Atezaz, Karlene Cunningham, and Richard M. Bloch. 2019. Depression and Anxiety Disorders: Benefits of Exercise, Yoga, and Meditation. *American Family Physician* 99: 620–27.

Schuch, Felipe B., Davy Vancampfort, Justin Richards, Simon Rosenbaum, Philip B. Ward, and Brendon Stubbs. 2016. Exercise as a treatment for depression: A meta-analysis adjusting for publication bias. *Journal of Psychiatric Research* 77: 42–51. [CrossRef]

Serafini, Gianluca, Bianca Parmigiani, Andrea Amerio, Andrea Aguglia, Leo Sher, and Mario Amore. 2020. The psychological impact of COVID-19 on the mental health in the general population. *QJM An International Journal of Medicine* 113: 531–37. [CrossRef]

Shimizu, Kazuhiro, Fuminori Kimura, Takayuki Akimoto, Takao Akama, Kai Tanabe, Takahiko Nishijima, Shinya Kuno, and Ichiro Kono. 2008. Effect of moderate exercise training on T-helper cell subpopulations in elderly people. *Exercise Immunology Review* 14: 24–37.

Song, Qing-Hua, Guo-Qing Shen, Rong-Mei Xu, Quan-Hai Zhang, Ming Ma, Yan-Hua Guo, Xin-Ping Zhao, and Yu-Bing Han. 2014. Effect of Tai Chi exercise on the physical and mental health of the elder patients suffered from anxiety disorder. *International Journal of Physiology, Pathophysiology and Pharmacology* 6: 55–60. [PubMed]

Stebbing, Justin, Anne Phelan, Ivan Griffin, Catherine Tucker, Olly Oechsle, Dan Smith, and Peter Richardson. 2020. COVID-19: Combining antiviral and anti-inflammatory treatments. *The Lancet Infectious Diseases* 20: 400–2. [CrossRef]

Stefan, Norbert, Andreas L. Birkenfeld, Matthias B. Schulze, and David S. Ludwig. 2020. Obesity and impaired metabolic health in patients with COVID-19. *Nature Reviews Endocrinology* 16: 341–42. [CrossRef]

Stonerock, Gregory L., Benson M. Hoffman, Patrick J. Smith, and James A. Blumenthal. 2015. Exercise as Treatment for Anxiety: Systematic Review and Analysis. *Annals of Behavioral Medicine* 49: 542–56. [CrossRef]

Stranahan, Alexis M., Kim Lee, and Mark P. Mattson. 2008. Central Mechanisms of HPA Axis Regulation by Voluntary Exercise. *Neuromolecular Medicine* 10: 118–27. [CrossRef]

Ströhle, Andreas. 2009. Physical activity, exercise, depression and anxiety disorders. *Journal of Neural Transmission* 116: 777–84. [CrossRef]

Stubbs, Brendon, Davy Vancampfort, Simon Rosenbaum, Joseph Firth, Theodore Cosco, Nicola Veronese, Giovanni A. Salum, and Felipe B. Schuch. 2017. An examination of the anxiolytic effects of exercise for people with anxiety and stress-related disorders: A meta-analysis. *Psychiatry Research* 249: 102–8. [CrossRef]

Tan, Tricia, Bernard Khoo, Edouard G. Mills, Maria Phylactou, Bijal Patel, Pei C. Eng, and Layla Thurston. 2020. Association between high serum total cortisol concentrations and mortality from COVID-19. *Lancet Diabetes Endocrinology* 8: 659–60. [CrossRef]

Vanuytsel, Tim, Sander Van Wanrooy, Hanne Vanheel, Christophe Vanormelingen, Sofie Verschueren, Els Houben, Shadea Salim Rasoel, J. Tóth, L. Holvoet, R. Farré, and et al. 2014. Psychological stress and corticotropin-releasing hormone increase intestinal permeability in humans by a mast cell-dependent mechanism. *Gut* 63: 1293–99. [CrossRef] [PubMed]

Vogelzangs, N., A. T. F. Beekman, P. De Jonge, and B. W. J. H. Penninx. 2013. Anxiety disorders and inflammation in a large adult cohort. *Translational Psychiatry* 3: e249. [CrossRef] [PubMed]

Wang, Meizi, Julien S. Baker, Wenjing Quan, Siqin Shen, Gusztáv Fekete, and Yaodong Gu. 2020. A Preventive Role of Exercise Across the Coronavirus 2 (SARS-CoV-2) Pandemic. *Frontiers in Physiology* 11: 572718. [CrossRef] [PubMed]

Wang, Minghuan, Caihong Hu, Qian Zhao, Renjie Feng, Qing Wang, Hongbin Cai, and Zhenli Guo. 2021. Acute psychological impact on COVID-19 patients in Hubei: A multicenter observational study. *Translational Psychiatry* 11: 133. [CrossRef] [PubMed]

World Health Organisation. 2021. Available online: https://www.who.int/emergencies/diseases/novel-coronavirus-2019 (accessed on 15 September 2021).

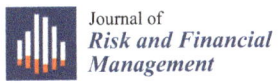

Journal of
Risk and Financial Management

Article

Behavioral and Mental Responses towards the COVID-19 Pandemic among Chinese Older Adults: A Cross-Sectional Study

Wei Liang [1,2], Yanping Duan [1,2,3,*], Min Yang [2], Borui Shang [4], Chun Hu [5], Yanping Wang [2] and Julien Steven Baker [1,2]

1. Center for Health and Exercise Science Research, Hong Kong Baptist University, Hong Kong 999077, China; wliang1020@hkbu.edu.hk (W.L.); jsbaker@hkbu.edu.hk (J.S.B.)
2. Department of Sport, Physical Education and Health, Hong Kong Baptist University, Hong Kong 999077, China; myanhkbu@gmail.com (M.Y.); yanniswyp@163.com (Y.W.)
3. College of Health Sciences, Wuhan Institute of Physical Education, Wuhan 430000, China
4. Department of Kinesiology, Hebei Institute of Physical Education, Shijiazhuang 050000, China; boruishang@hepec.edu.cn
5. Student Mental Health Education Center, Northwestern Polytechnical University, Xi'an 710000, China; huchun52@163.com
* Correspondence: duanyp@hkbu.edu.hk

Citation: Liang, Wei, Yanping Duan, Min Yang, Borui Shang, Chun Hu, Yanping Wang, and Julien Steven Baker. 2021. Behavioral and Mental Responses towards the COVID-19 Pandemic among Chinese Older Adults: A Cross-Sectional Study. *Journal of Risk and Financial Management* 14: 568. https://doi.org/10.3390/jrfm14120568

Academic Editor: Thanasis Stengos

Received: 1 October 2021
Accepted: 16 November 2021
Published: 24 November 2021

Publisher's Note: MDPI stays neutral with regard to jurisdictional claims in published maps and institutional affiliations.

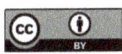

Copyright: © 2021 by the authors. Licensee MDPI, Basel, Switzerland. This article is an open access article distributed under the terms and conditions of the Creative Commons Attribution (CC BY) license (https://creativecommons.org/licenses/by/4.0/).

Abstract: The novel COVID-19 pandemic spread quickly and continuously influenced global societies. As a vulnerable population that accounted for the highest percentage of deaths from the pandemic, older adults have experienced huge life-altering challenges and increased risks of mental problems during the pandemic. Empirical evidence is needed to develop effective strategies to promote preventive measures and mitigate the adverse psychological impacts of the COVID-19 pandemic. This study aimed to investigate the behavioral responses (i.e., preventive behaviors, physical activity, fruit and vegetable consumption) and mental responses (i.e., depression and loneliness) towards the COVID-19 pandemic among Chinese older adults. A further aim was to identify the associations among demographics, behavioral responses, and mental responses. Using a convenience sampling approach, 516 older adults were randomly recruited from five cities of Hubei province in China. Results of the cross-sectional survey showed that 11.7% of participants did not adhere to the WHO recommended preventive measures, while 37.6% and 8.3% of participants decreased physical activity and fruit–vegetable consumption respectively. For mental responses, 30.8% and 69.2% of participants indicated significantly depressive symptoms and severe loneliness, respectively. Participants' behavioral and mental responses differed significantly in several demographics, such as age group, living situation, marital status, education levels, household income, medical conditions, and perceived health status. Demographic correlates and behavioral responses could significantly predicate the mental response with small-to-moderate effect sizes. This is the first study to investigate the characteristics of behavioral and mental responses of Chinese older adults during the COVID-19 pandemic. Research findings may give new insights into future developments of effective interventions and policies to promote health among older adults in the fight against the pandemic.

Keywords: COVID-19; preventive behaviors; physical activity (PA); fruit and vegetable consumption (FVC); depression; loneliness; older adults; China; behavioral response; mental response

1. Introduction

The novel coronavirus disease (COVID-19) has continuously influenced global societies, causing over 219 million confirmed cases and 4.55 million deaths as reported on 25 September 2021 by the World Health Organization (WHO 2021a). In China, there have been more than 96,000 confirmed cases and over 4600 fatality cases to date (National Health Commission of China 2021; CSSE 2021). As a vulnerable group, older adults have accounted for the highest proportion of deaths from COVID-19 (approximately 75%)

(Shahid et al. 2020; World Health Organization 2020). During the COVID-19 pandemic, healthy ageing advocacy is being confronted with a great challenge.

To reduce the human-to-human transmission of the coronavirus, many countries enacted the emergent lockdown policy and implemented strict control measures for the pandemic (Cheng et al. 2020; Hu et al. 2021). For example, in China, the government of Hubei Wuhan imposed an urgent lockdown on 23 January 2020, with travel restrictions. Despite the positive effects in preventing the spread of the pandemic, these governmental actions have led to great life-altering challenges for individuals especially for older adults, e.g., the routinization of practicing preventive behaviors (PB) in daily life, and huge changes in physical activity (PA), and dietary behavior, e.g., fruit-and-vegetable consumption (FVC) (Li et al. 2020; Dwyer et al. 2020; Weaver et al. 2021).

In addition to the lifestyle changes, older adults have a high risk of psychological distress during the pandemic. Compared with other age groups, older adults are more likely to experience fear of becoming ill or dying during the pandemic, which may be accompanied by feelings of helplessness and stigma (Khan et al. 2020; Vahia et al. 2020). These feelings can lead to a series of negative mental responses and problems, such as loneliness and depression, consequently imposing adverse influences on the overall health and well-being of older adults (Khan et al. 2020; Vahia et al. 2020; Singh and Singh 2020). This will also impose a series of negative impacts on diverse aspects of society, such as burdening the medical systems and affecting the success in the labor market (Codagnone et al. 2020; Usher et al. 2020). Older adults' behavioral and mental responses during the pandemic not only provides useful information for health risk communication and pandemic prevention but also contributes to achieving the advocacy of healthy ageing.

2. Literature Review

Individuals' behavioral responses during the pandemic usually include three major aspects: PB adherence, PA change, and dietary change (e.g., FVC) (Weaver et al. 2021; Puspitasari et al. 2020; Balkhi et al. 2020). Individual precautionary actions, such as hand washing, facemask wearing, and physical distancing, which are recommended by the WHO and other health authority organizations (World Health Organization 2020; Probst et al. 2020), have become individual's daily routines. An overwhelming amount of evidence has demonstrated that adhering to these three PB could effectively inhibit the transmission of COVID-19 and reduce the probability of infection (Probst et al. 2020). Several studies have examined the practice of PB among populations from diverse countries and regions (Arora and Grey 2020; Ye et al. 2020). For example, a review study summarized the knowledge, attitude, and practice of PB during the pandemic among healthcare workers, medical students, and populations in the US, the UK, Italy, Jordan, and China in the initial stage of the pandemic (Arora and Grey 2020). Some empirical studies also investigated the PB adherence among adults and internet users in China (Li and Liu 2020; Ye et al. 2020). However, there is limited evidence particularly targeting the characteristics of PB adherence among older adults, especially in China. For PA and FVC, a recent review summarized the results of 41 studies finding that most of the evidence identified a decrease in PA levels during the pandemic, whereas only one study targeted community-dwelling older adults (Caputo and Reichert 2020). Several studies have investigated the FVC behavior among children and adults, while evidence for Chinese older adults is still limited (López-Bueno et al. 2020; Litton and Beavers 2020).

Behavioral responses have been evident to impose considerable influences on individuals' mental health outcomes/responses. For example, recent studies have indicated an inverse association of adhering to PB with mental distress among adolescents and adults (Wang et al. 2020; Cunningham et al. 2020; Gehlich et al. 2019). This may generate urgently needed insights into the mitigation of negative mental impacts of the pandemic. Nevertheless, there are few studies examining the impact of adhering to PB on mental health outcomes among older adults. For PA and FVC, as a common healthy lifestyle pattern, they also play an irreplaceable role in the battle with the COVID-19 pandemic, as through engaging in regular PA and consuming sufficient FVC individuals could enhance their cardiorespiratory fitness and immune function, as a result reducing the risk of death from viral infection (Amatriain-Fernández et al. 2020; Yahia et al. 2017). However, self-isolation and restrictions during the pandemic dramatically reduced the opportunities for individuals to be physical active and increase the possibilities of unhealthy diets (e.g., insufficient FVC). These unfavorable behavioral changes may lead to adverse mental consequences, e.g., worsening loneliness and depression, among older adults. Investigating the impact of such behavioral responses towards the pandemic in older adults should be prioritized. To the best of our knowledge, few studies have examined the relationship between all three behavioral responses (PB adherence, PA, and FVC) and mental responses (loneliness and depression) among older adults during the COVID-19 pandemic.

Given the lack of empirical research in China, the current study aimed to (1) investigate the demographic characteristics of behavioral (i.e., PB, PA, and FVC) and mental responses (i.e., loneliness and depressive symptoms) among Chinese older adults, and (2) examine the interrelationships between demographics, behavioral responses, and mental responses among Chinese older adults.

3. Materials and Methods

3.1. Study Design and Participants

To address the above objectives, this study used a cross-sectional design, and the data was collected from 15 June to 10 July 2020 (the lockdown had been withdrawn for over two months) with a convenience sampling approach. The sample size was calculated using G*Power 3.1 software. For achieving a medium effect size (Cohen's $f^2 = 0.15$) on the prediction of demographics and behavioral correlates in mental responses based on previous studies with older adults (Pinquart 2001), with an alpha of 0.05, a statistical power of 80%, and a response rate of 60%, a total of 205 participants were required. As shown in Figure 1, we contacted 727 participants and received an 83.8% response rate. Finally, 516 participants were included in data analysis. The eligible criteria included (1) older adults who are ≥ 60 years old; (2) not having been infected with COVID-19; (3) not having any cognitive disorders or impairments; (4) having access to a mobile phone or laptop; and (5) having sufficient reading or listening skills in Mandarin. For participants who have difficulties in using mobile phones or laptops, their family members or friends were invited to assist them in completing the online survey. The study was implemented and reported following the guidelines of the STROBE checklist.

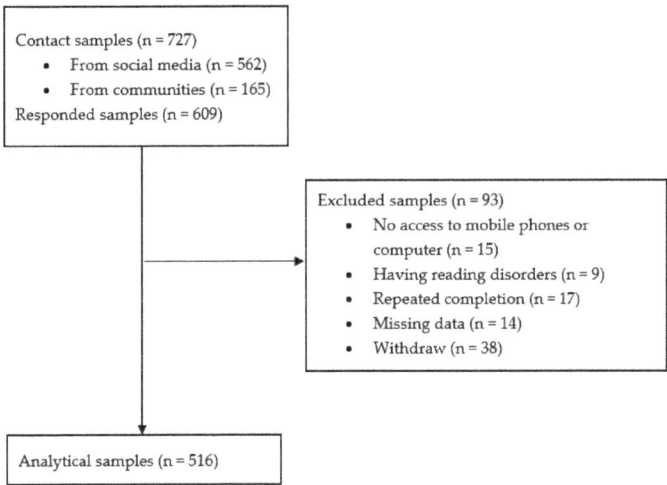

Figure 1. Flow diagram of participant recruitment.

3.2. Procedure

The questionnaire survey was administered using an online survey platform, namely SOJUMP (Changsha Ranxing Information Technology Co., Ltd., Changsha, China). The recruitment information was delivered by different social media channels, such as WeChat, Weibo, and QQ which are popular in China. In addition to the social media channels, researchers contacted the administration staff in several universities and neighborhood communities to facilitate recruitment to retired colleagues.

The duration of completing the online survey was about 15–20 minutes. To increase the engagement of participation, each participant who completed the questionnaires was provided with 30 RMB incentive by electronic transfer via WeChat or Alipay or by prepaid telephone recharge. All participants were asked to sign an informed consent form on the first page of the survey website prior to filling in the questionnaires. Ethical approval for the study was obtained from the Research Ethics Committee of Hong Kong Baptist University (REC/19-20/0490).

3.3. Measures

3.3.1. Behavioral Responses

- Preventive behaviors (PB): the adherence to the PB was measured by six items covering the three major PB as recommended by the WHO, including hand washing, facemask wearing, and physical distancing (WHO 2021b). Each behavior was assessed by two items. For example, the items for hand washing were asked with the stem of "during the previous week, I adhered to washing my hands with soap and water or alcohol-based hand rub (for at least 20 s, on all surfaces of the hands) ... " followed by two situations including "(a) in a daily life situation, e.g., before eating, and (b) in a disease-related situation, e.g., after caring for the sick." All responses were indicated on a 4-point Likert scale ranging from "1 = strongly disagree" to "4 = strongly agree" (Liang et al. 2021). Participants who indicated "agree/strongly agree" for all six items were coded as "1 = adhering to PB", otherwise as "0 = non-adhering to PB".
- Physical activity (PA) and fruit–vegetable consumption (FVC): each behavior response was measured by one item. Participants were asked about their changes in weekly amount of PA and daily portion of FVC since the outbreak of the COVID-19 pandemic. Responses included "0 = less" and "1 = same or more".

3.3.2. Mental Responses

- Depression: the 10-item Chinese version of the Epidemiologic Studies Short Depression Scale (CESD-10) was used to measure the depressive symptoms (Rankin et al. 1993). The questions were asked with the stem: "In the past week, how often I feel...", followed by 10 items such as "I was bothered by things that usually don't bother me". The responses were indicated on a 4-point Likert scale, ranging from "0 = rarely (less than 1 day)" to "3 = for most of the time (5–7 days)" (Cronbach's alpha = 0.82) (Rankin et al. 1993; Liang et al. 2019). The total score of the 10 items was calculated, where the score of 0–9 was coded as "0 = no significant depressive symptoms", and ≥ 10 was coded as "1 = significant depressive symptoms" (Andresen et al. 1994).
- Loneliness: the 6-item Chinese version of the De Jong Grieveld Loneliness Scale was used to measure loneliness (Leung et al. 2008). The scale consisted of two dimensions (social lonely and emotional lonely), with three items for each dimension. Participants were asked with the stem "Please see if the statements are describing your situations or feelings now ... " followed by six items, such as "I experience a general sense of emptiness" (emotional) and "There are plenty of people I can rely on when I have problems" (social) (Cronbach's alpha = 0.76) (Leung et al. 2008). The total score of the 6 items was calculated, where the score of 0–3 was coded as "0 = light loneliness" and ≥ 4 was coded as "1 = severe loneliness" (De Jong Gierveld and Van Tilburg 1999).

3.3.3. Demographics

Demographic information included age, gender, living situation, marital status, educational level, occupational status, household income, perceived health status, and medical condition.

3.4. Statistical Analysis

Data analyses were conducted using the IBM SPSS 26.0 (Armonk, NY, USA). Mean values, standard deviation (SD), and percentage (%) were calculated for descriptive analyses. The characteristics of behavioral and mental responses were examined using Chi-square tests. Single level and multi-level logistic regression models were used to explore the association among demographics, behavioral responses, and mental responses. The statistical significance was set at 0.05 (two-tailed). The effect sizes (Cohen's f^2) of association in the regression models were calculated using the formula "$f^2 = R^2/(1-R^2)$", with 0.02, 0.15, and 0.35 indicating a small, medium, and large effect, respectively (Selya et al. 2012; Duan et al. 2021).

4. Results

4.1. Characteristics of the Study Sample

A total of 516 eligible participants (57.9% females) were included in data analysis, ranging in age from 60 to 90 years old (Mean $_{age}$ = 67.6 ± 6.6 yrs.). Over 90% of participants lived with others (e.g., spouse or children) and more than 80% of participants were married. In total, 44.8% of participants received middle or high school education, while the percentage of participants receiving college or above education was 46.5%. Most participants were pensioners or retired (92.6%), and over half of participants reported an average level of household income (57.9%). For the medical condition, 50.8% of participants had a history of chronic diseases. More than half of participants perceived their health status as good (52.7%). Details can be found in Table 1.

Table 1. Characteristics of the study sample, behavioral responses, and mental responses (n = 516).

	PB	PA	FVC	Depression	Loneliness
	Non-Adherence: n (%)	Decreased: n (%)	Decreased: n (%)	Yes: n (%)	High: n (%)
Total (n = 516)					
Age (n, %)					
60–69 yrs. (354, 68.60%)	36 (10.2%)	125 (35.3%)	23 (6.5%) *	105 (29.7%)	233 (65.8%)
70–79 yrs. (128, 24.80%)	128 (11.7%)	52 (40.6%)	13 (10.2%) *	42 (32.8%)	76 (59.4%)
≥80 yrs. (34, 6.60%)	34 (11.8%)	17 (50.0%)	7 (20.6%) *	12 (35.3%)	18 (52.9%)
Gender (n, %)					
Male (217, 42.10%)	26 (12.0%)	77 (35.5%)	19 (8.8%)	69 (31.8%)	132 (60.8%)
Female (299, 57.90%)	29 (9.7%)	171 (39.1%)	24 (8.0%)	90 (30.1%)	195 (65.2%)
Living situation (n, %)					
Alone (48, 9.30%)	13 (27.1%) ***	20 (41.7%)	7 (14.6%)	21 (43.80%) *	29 (60.4%)
Not alone (468, 90.70%)	42 (9.0%) ***	174 (37.2%)	36 (7.7%)	138 (29.5%) *	298 (73.7%)
Marital status (n, %)					
Single (14, 2.70%)	3 (21.4%) *	7 (50.0%)	1 (7.1%)	5 (35.7%) **	10 (71.4%)
Married (432, 83.70%)	39 (9.0%) *	154 (35.6%)	33 (7.6%)	120 (27.8%) **	275 (63.7%)
Divorced/widowed (70, 13.60%)	13 (18.6%) *	33 (41.7%)	9 (12.9%)	34 (48.6%) **	42 (60.0%)
Educational level (n, %)					
Primary school or below (45, 8.70%)	12 (26.7%) ***	18 (40.0%)	5 (11.1%)	21 (46.7%) *	28 (62.2%)
Middle or High school (231, 44.80%)	29 (12.6%) ***	81 (35.1%)	21 (9.1%)	74 (32.0%) *	149 (64.5%)
College or above (240, 46.50%)	14 (5.8%) ***	95 (39.6%)	17 (7.1%)	64 (26.7%) *	150 (62.5%)
Occupational status (n, %)					
Employed (16, 3.10%)	3 (18.8%)	2 (12.5%)	0 (0.00%)	4 (20.5%)	11 (68.8%)
Pensioner or retired (478, 92.60%)	47 (9.8%)	186 (38.9%)	40 (8.4%)	146 (30.5%)	303 (63.4%)
Unemployed (22, 4.30%)	5 (9.10%)	6 (27.3%)	3 (13.6%)	9 (40.9%)	13 (59.1%)

Table 1. Cont.

	PB	PA	FVC	Depression	Loneliness
	Non-Adherence: n (%)	Decreased: n (%)	Decreased: n (%)	Yes: n (%)	High: n (%)
Household income (n, %)					
Below average (113, 21.90%)	21 (18.6%) **	43 (38.1%)	10 (8.8%)	48 (42.5%) **	69 (61.1%)
Average (299, 57.90%)	28 (9.4%) **	108 (36.1%)	24 (8.0%)	89 (29.8%) **	191 (63.9%)
Above average (104, 20.20%)	6 (5.8%) **	43 (41.3%)	9 (8.7%)	22 (21.2%) **	67 (64.4%)
Health status (n, %)					
Poor (48, 9.30%)	6 (12.5%)	21 (43.80%)	5 (10.4%)	28 (58.3%) ***	25 (52.1%)
Satisfactory (196, 38.00%)	24 (12.20%)	84 (42.90%)	19 (9.7%)	69 (35.2%) ***	119 (60.7%)
Excellent (272, 52.70%)	25 (9.2%)	89 (32.7%)	19 (7.0%)	62 (22.8%) ***	183 (67.3%)
Medical condition (n, %)					
No (254, 49.20%)	28 (11.0%)	83 (32.7%) *	16 (6.3%)	66 (26.0%) *	167 (65.7%)
Yes (262, 50.80%)	27 (10.3%)	111 (42.4%) *	27 (10.3%)	93 (35.5%) *	160 (61.1%)

Note. PB = preventive behaviors; PA = physical activity; FVC = fruit and vegetable consumption; *** $p < 0.001$, ** $p < 0.01$, * $p < 0.05$.

4.2. Characteristics of Behavioral and Mental Responses

As shown in Table 1, 11.7% of participants did not comply with the recommended PB in response to the COVID-19 pandemic, while since the outbreak of the pandemic 37.6% and 8.3% of participants decreased their weekly amount of PA and daily portion of FVC, respectively. For mental responses, 30.8% of participants had significant depressive symptoms, while 69.2% of participants felt lonely.

Participants' behavioral responses differed significantly in a series of demographics. In particular, the compliance with PB was significantly poorer for participants who lived alone ($p = 0.001$), who were single or divorced/windowed ($p = 0.023$), received no or primary education ($p < 0.001$), and had lower household incomes ($p = 0.005$). For PA, a significantly higher percentage of participants with decreasing PA was found among those who had medical histories of chronic diseases (e.g., cardiovascular diseases, diabetes, cancer, and respiratory illness) ($p = 0.023$), while PA change did not differ significantly in other demographics ($p = 0.054$ to 0.634). For FVC, participants who were in the 70–79 yrs./$\geq$80 yrs. age groups showed a significantly higher percentage for reducing the daily FVC compared with those in the 60–69 yrs. group ($p = 0.012$).

Regarding mental responses, the proportion of participants showing significant depressive symptoms was significantly higher among those who lived alone ($p = 0.042$), who were single or divorced/windowed ($p = 0.002$), illiterate or only received primary education ($p = 0.025$), economic disadvantaged ($p = 0.003$), perceived bad health status ($p < 0.001$), and had a medical history of chronic diseases ($p = 0.019$). For loneliness, it did not differ significantly in any demographic variables ($p = 0.081$ to 0.891).

4.3. Associations of Demographic Correlates, Behavioral Responses, and Mental Responses

As shown in Table 2, a series of binary logistic regression models were conducted to explore the association between demographics and behavioral responses among participants. For PB, results showed that PB non-adherence was significantly associated with living situation (OR = 0.31, 95%CI = 0.12 to 0.79, $p = 0.014$) and education levels (OR = 0.20, 95%CI = 0.07 to 0.59, $p = 0.003$). None of the demographic variables were statistically associated with PA change ($p = 0.098$ to 0.958). For FVC, participants who were in the $\geq$80 yrs. age group were more likely to decrease the daily portion of FVC compared with those in the younger age group (60–69 yrs.) (OR = 2.85, 95%CI = 1.02 to 7.95, $p = 0.045$).

Table 2. Associations of demographics and behavioral responses ($n = 516$).

Variable	PB Non-Adherence		PA Decrease		FVC Decrease	
	OR	95%CI	OR	95%CI	OR	95%CI
Age group (60–69 yrs. as ref.)						
70–79 yrs.	0.82	(0.40, 1.71)	1.08	(0.69, 1.67)	1.30	(0.62, 2.75)
≥80 yrs.	0.74	(0.22, 2.55)	1.55	(0.73, 3.31)	2.85 *	(1.02, 7.95)
Gender (male as ref.)						
Female	0.58	(0.31, 1.09)	1.10	(0.75, 1.63)	0.84	(0.43, 1.64)
Living situation (alone as ref.)						
Not alone	0.31	(0.12, 0.79)	1.19	(0.58, 2.42)	0.58	(0.20, 1.68)
Marital status (single as ref.)						
Married	0.36	(0.08, 1.64)	0.56	(0.18, 1.72)	0.97	(0.11, 8.34)
Divorced/widowed	0.38	(0.08, 1.96)	0.91	(0.27, 3.05)	1.25	(0.13, 11.68)
Educational level (primary school or below as ref.)						
Middle or high school	0.49	(0.19, 1.26)	0.84	(0.39, 1.80)	1.29	(0.38, 4.39)
College or above	0.20 **	(0.07, 0.59)	1.00	(0.46, 2.19)	0.98	(0.27, 3.64)
Occupational status (employed as ref.)						
Unemployed	0.47	(0.11, 2.08)	3.62	(0.79, 16.57)	N/A	N/A
Pensioner or retired	0.45	(0.07, 3.07)	1.96	(0.31, 12.53)	N/A	N/A
Household income (below above as ref.)						
Average	0.62	(0.31, 1.24)	0.99	(0.61, 1.60)	1.12	(0.49, 2.58)
Above average	0.43	(0.15, 1.28)	1.21	(0.66, 2.24)	1.25	(0.43, 3.66)
Health status (poor as ref.)						
Satisfactory	1.40	(0.47, 4.21)	1.05	(0.53, 2.06)	1.21	(0.40, 3.66)
Excellent	0.89	(0.28, 2.86)	0.77	(0.38, 1.56)	1.09	(0.34, 3.47)
Medical condition (no chronic diseases as ref.)						
Yes	0.80	(0.41, 1.56)	1.29	(0.86, 1.94)	1.56	(0.76, 3.19)

Note. PB = preventive behaviors; PA = physical activity; FVC = fruit and vegetable consumption; N/A = not applicable: the statistical analysis could not be conducted due to the unbalanced data distribution; ** $p < 0.01$, * $p < 0.05$.

As presented in Table 3, multi-level binary logistic regression models were employed to examine the association of mental responses with demographic correlates and behavioral responses. In Model 1, participants who perceived satisfactory (OR = 0.42, 95%CI = 0.21 to 0.84, $p = 0.014$) and excellent (OR = 0.23, 95%CI = 0.11 to 0.48, $p < 0.001$) health status were less likely to indicate significant depressive symptoms compared with those who reported bad health status. In Model 2, after controlling for the demographics, depression was found to be significantly and positively associated with both decreased FVC (OR = 2.77, 95%CI = 1.35 to 5.69, $p = 0.006$) and non-adherence of PB (OR = 2.84, 95%CI = 1.51 to 5.33, $p = 0.001$). The entire model of demographics and behavioral correlates showed a moderate effect size for explaining the variance in participants' depressive symptoms (Cohen's $f^2 = 0.22$).

For loneliness, there were no statistically significant associations between demographic correlates and loneliness ($p = 0.189$ to 0.973) in Model 1. After controlling for demographics, a significantly positive associated was found between decreased PA and severe loneliness (OR = 2.01, 95%CI = 1.32 to 3.05, $p = 0.001$) in Model 2. The entire model of demographics and behavioral correlates showed a small effect size for explaining the variance in participants' loneliness (Cohen's $f^2 = 0.06$). The zero-order Spearman correlation matrix can be found in Appendix A.

Table 3. Associations of demographics and behavioral responses with mental responses ($n = 516$).

Variable	Depression				Loneliness			
	Model 1		Model 2		Model 1		Model 2	
	OR	95%CI	OR	95%CI	OR	95%CI	OR	95%CI
Age group (60–69 yrs. as ref.)								
70–79 yrs.	0.83	(0.52, 1.35)	0.82	(0.50, 1.35)	0.81	(0.52, 1.26)	0.81	(0.52, 1.26)
≥80 yrs.	0.74	(0.32, 1.75)	0.64	(0.26, 1.47)	0.65	(0.30, 1.38)	0.63	(0.29, 1.36)
Gender (male as ref.)								
Female	0.79	(0.52, 1.21)	0.84	(0.54, 1.29)	1.18	(0.80, 1.73)	1.15	(0.78, 1.70)
Living situation (alone as ref.)								
Not alone	0.86	(0.41, 1.80)	1.07	(0.49, 2.35)	1.08	(0.53, 2.20)	1.00	(0.48, 2.07)
Marital status (single as ref.)								
Married	0.73	(0.22, 2.51)	0.87	(0.24, 3.20)	0.67	(0.20, 2.27)	0.72	(0.21, 2.48)
Divorced/widowed	1.68	(0.45, 6.18)	1.98	(0.50, 7.89)	0.60	(0.17, 2.19)	0.59	(0.16, 2.21)
Educational level (primary school or below as ref.)								
Middle or high school	0.70	(0.32, 1.52)	0.75	(0.33, 1.69)	0.91	(0.43, 1.94)	0.94	(0.44, 2.00)
College or above	0.55	(0.25, 1.24)	0.64	(0.27, 1.50)	0.81	(0.37, 1.77)	0.79	(0.36, 1.73)
Occupational status (employed as ref.)								
Unemployed	0.89	(0.27, 2.97)	0.84	(0.24, 2.91)	0.93	(0.31, 2.81)	0.82	(0.27, 2.50)
Pensioner or retired	0.65	(0.13, 3.18)	0.59	(0.11, 3.06)	0.85	(0.20, 3.69)	0.84	(0.19, 3.70)
Household income (below above as ref.)								
Average	0.81	(0.50, 1.33)	0.83	(0.50, 1.39)	1.03	(0.64, 1.65)	1.02	(0.63, 1.66)
Above average	0.58	(0.30, 1.14)	0.59	(0.29, 1.17)	1.10	(0.60, 2.20)	1.07	(0.58, 1.97)
Health status (poor as ref.)								
Satisfactory	0.42 *	(0.21, 0.84)	0.37 **	(0.18, 0.76)	1.33	(0.68, 2.60)	1.35	(0.69, 2.66)
Excellent	0.23 ***	(0.11, 0.48)	0.21 ***	(0.10, 0.46)	1.71	(0.85, 3.44)	1.81	(0.89, 3.69)
Medical condition (no chronic diseases as ref.)								
Yes	1.10	(0.70, 1.72)	1.04	(0.65, 1.64)	1.00	(0.66, 1.50)	0.97	(0.64, 1.47)
PA (same and more as ref.)								
Decrease	N/A	N/A	1.39	(0.90, 2.15)	N/A	N/A	2.01 **	(1.32, 3.05)
FVC (same and more as ref.)								
Decrease	N/A	N/A	2.77 **	(1.35, 5.69)	N/A	N/A	0.62	(0.31, 1.23)
PB (adherence as ref.)								
Non-adherence	N/A	N/A	2.84 **	(1.51, 5.33)	N/A	N/A	0.82	(0.45, 1.52)

Note. PB = preventive behaviors; PA = physical activity; FVC = fruit and vegetable consumption; N/A = not applicable; *** $p < 0.001$, ** $p < 0.01$, * $p < 0.05$.

5. Discussion

This is the first online cross-sectional study to comprehensively explore the characteristics of behavioral responses (PB, PA, and FVC) and mental responses (depression and loneliness) towards the COVID-19 pandemic among Chinese older adults. Non-negligible percentages of Chinese older adults showed negative behavioral responses (i.e., non-adherence to PB, decreased PA and FVC) during the pandemic, while the mental responses were alarming. For older adults' behavioral responses, PB, PA, and FVC were found to differ significantly in diverse demographics. For older adults' mental responses, only depression differed significantly in demographics, while loneliness did show specific patterns. Age group, living situation, and education levels were significantly associated with PB and FVC. After controlling for demographics, there were significant associations found between behavioral responses and loneliness among Chinese older adults.

Our research findings have identified demographic differences in both behavioral and mental responses among the study sample, suggesting that future intervention development and policy making should take the participants' demographic characteristics into consideration. For the behavioral responses, despite the relevant legal penalties and mass information campaigns, we found there were still few older adults who did not comply with the recommended PB. Consistent with other studies, the percentage of older adults non-adhering to PB was not high (Ye et al. 2020); however, there is still a need to promote the adoption of PB in response to the pandemic among older adults especially due to the high vulnerability and severity of this population (Singh and Singh 2020). For PA, it is not surprising that more than 35% of older adults decreased their weekly PA. This finding is consistent with other empirical evidence, where the decreased PA may be attributed to both governmental policy (e.g., closure of parks, gyms, or sport centers) and fear of infection while doing exercise outside (Hu et al. 2020; Qin et al. 2020; Wilczyńska et al. 2021; Schrack et al. 2020). For FVC, most older adults maintained or increased the fruit and vegetable consumption, where similar findings have been also reported in previous studies. Based on psychological theories of behavior change (e.g., social cognition theory), we conclude that the governmental efforts (e.g., increase the supply of food after the lockdown) social support, and older adults' heath knowledge and belief, may play an important role in maintaining and increasing nutritional food consumption (Anderson et al. 2007). This assumption needs to be further examined especially within the pandemic context in future research. Overall, the findings of behavioral responses highlight the need of more supportive measures to promote the adherence of PB and facilitate the adoption of healthy lifestyle behaviors during the pandemics (e.g., governmental welfare, behavior promotion campaigns, education workshops). For the mental responses, consistent with previous evidence, the situation of older adults' mental problems was alarming during the pandemic (Yang et al. 2020; Wu 2020; Wang et al. 2020). This highlights an urgent need of mental healthcare services for older adults during the COVID-19 and future pandemics (Wu 2020).

For the associations among demographics, behavioral responses, and mental responses, we found that the older adults who lived alone and had lower education levels were more likely to not comply with the PB in response to the pandemic, while older adults who were older were more likely to decrease the daily FVC. Consistent with previous studies, these findings emphasized the importance and necessity of caring for the social disadvantaged sample, e.g., enhancing the social and governmental support, organizing educational workshops (Shankar et al. 2010; Li et al. 2020). In line with previous studies, we found that older adults who did not adhere to PB and decreased daily FVC were more likely to show significant depressive symptoms, while those who decreased weekly PA were more likely to show severe loneliness (Wang et al. 2020; Stickley et al. 2020; Kingsbury et al. 2016; Pels and Kleinert 2016). These findings emphasize the importance of promoting positive behavioral responses (e.g., comply with PB, perform healthy lifestyles) among older adults during the pandemic, with the aim to promote their mental well-being and overall health. Our findings also demonstrate implications for the economy aspects. Particularly given the large healthcare (USD 0.62 billion) and societal costs (USD 383.02 billion) related to the COVID-19 pandemic (Jin et al. 2021), promoting such positive behavioral responses will be beneficial not only for mitigating the adverse physical and mental impacts of the pandemic towards individuals, but also for lessening the huge burden on healthcare systems in terms of hospitalization, medication, staff, and equipment for critical care costs.

Despite the implications of this study, several limitations need to be considered. First, due to the convenience sampling and the use of online questionnaire survey, the participants may vary in relation to the actual patterns of the general older adults. More empirical studies with a larger sample size using random stratified sampling are needed in the future to enhance the representativeness and external validity. Moreover, the data was obtained from a specific age group from Hubei province in China; therefore, it is unclear whether these findings could be generalized to other age groups and different cultural contexts. Furthermore, the use of self-reported scales might lead to recall bias, self-perception bias, and social desirability effects (Liu et al. 2021). Additionally, PA and FVC used one item in the study which might influence the accuracy of measuring target outcomes and applying comprehensive questionnaires to measure these variables is warranted in future studies. Finally, the causal relationship and underlying mechanisms of the associations could be identified in this study due to the use of cross-sectional design and without inclusion of some theory-based psychosocial determinants. More research on this issue is warranted.

6. Conclusions

The current study investigated the characteristics of Chinese older adults' behavioral and mental responses towards the COVID-19 pandemic and examined the interrelationships among demographics, behavioral responses, and mental responses among Chinese older adults. Older adults' behavioral responses differed significantly in diverse demographics, such as age group, living situation, marital status, education levels, household income, and medical condition, while in terms of mental responses, only depressive symptoms differed significantly in several demographics, yet older adults' loneliness did not show any special characteristics. The findings revealed the importance of considering different demographics when designing interventions and making relevant policies in the fight against the pandemic. Older adults' negative mental responses were significantly associated with negative behavioral responses, suggesting the need and necessity of developing more health behavior promotion programs for mitigating the negative impacts of the pandemic and for achieving the long-term advocacy of healthy aging. Overall, our findings may add value to research and practice of promoting health among older adults during COVID-19 and future pandemics. Further studies that use a stricter scientific design with a larger sample size and objective measures that examine psychological mechanisms with inclusion of theory-based constructs are warranted in the future.

Author Contributions: Conceptualization, Y.D. and W.L.; methodology, W.L., Y.D., B.S. and C.H.; software, W.L. and M.Y.; validation, Y.D., W.L. and C.H.; formal analysis, M.Y. and W.L.; investigation, all authors; resources, all authors; data curation, Y.D., W.L. and M.Y.; writing—original draft preparation, W.L.; writing—review and editing, J.S.B.; project administration, Y.D.; funding acquisition, Y.D. All authors have read and agreed to the published version of the manuscript.

Funding: This research was funded by the Start-Up Grant and Strategic Development Fund (SDF) of Hong Kong Baptist University (HKBU). The funding organization had no role in the study design, study implementation, data collection, data analysis, manuscript preparation, or publication decision. The work is the responsibility of the authors. The APC was funded by the conference "Transnational and Transdisciplinary Lessons from the Covid-19 Pandemic", an International Symposium Organized by the Department of Government and International Studies in association, HKBU with the Department of Sport, Physical Education and Health, HKBU and the David C Lam Institute for East-West Studies.

Institutional Review Board Statement: The study was conducted according to the guidelines of the Declaration of Helsinki, and approved by the Research Ethics Committee of Hong Kong Baptist University (REC/19-20/0490).

Informed Consent Statement: Informed consent was obtained from all subjects involved in the study.

Data Availability Statement: Available from the corresponding author on reasonable request.

Acknowledgments: We would like to express our gratitude to all the contributions made by the researchers who were involved in the project.

Conflicts of Interest: The authors declare no conflict of interest.

Appendix A

Table A1. Spearman correlation matrix of study variables.

	1	2	3	4	5	6	7	8	9	10	11	12	13
1. Age	1.000												
2. Gender	−0.035												
3. Living situation	−0.140 **	−0.124 **											
4. Marital status	0.143 **	0.123 **	−0.370 **										
5. Education level	−0.150 **	−0.139 **	0.064	−0.175 **									
6. Occupation	0.151 **	0.079	−0.060	0.155 **	−0.241 **								
7. Household Income	0.011	−0.022	0.115 **	−0.133 **	0.295 **	−0.153 **							
8. Health status	−0.190 **	0.010	0.012	−0.009	0.040	−0.138 **	0.172 **						
9. Medical condition	0.170 **	−0.046	−0.022	−0.003	0.052	−0.030	−0.063	−0.418 **					
10. PB adherence	0.023	−0.037	−0.170 **	0.069	−0.174 **	0.032	−0.136 **	−0.049	−0.012				
11. PA change	0.076	0.037	−0.027	0.054	0.029	0.025	0.021	−0.104 *	0.100 *	0.043			
12. FVC change	0.110 *	−0.013	−0.072	0.061	−0.046	0.065	−0.003	−0.052	0.072	0.032	0.287 **		
13. Depression	0.038	−0.018	−0.090 *	0.130 **	−0.104 *	0.049	−0.151 **	−0.212 **	0.103 *	0.191 **	0.132 **	0.163 **	
14. Loneliness	−0.079	0.045	0.020	−0.036	−0.013	−0.027	0.023	0.095 *	−0.049	−0.024	0.117 **	−0.033	−0.015

Note. PB = preventive behaviors; PA = physical activity; FVC = fruit and vegetable consumption. ** $p < .01$, * $p < .05$.

References

Amatriain-Fernández, Sandra, Eric Simón Murillo-Rodríguez, Thomas Gronwald, Sergio Machado, and Henning Budde. 2020. Benefits of physical activity and physical exercise in the time of pandemic. *Psychological Trauma: Theory, Research, Practice, and Policy* 12: S264. [CrossRef] [PubMed]

Anderson, Eileen S., Richard A. Winett, and Janet R. Wojcik. 2007. Self-regulation, self-efficacy, outcome expectations, and social support: Social cognitive theory and nutrition behavior. *Annals of Behavioral Medicine* 34: 304–12. [CrossRef] [PubMed]

Andresen, Elena M., Judith A. Malmgren, William B. Carter, and Donald L. Patrick. 1994. Screening for depression in well older adults: Evaluation of a short form of the CES-D. *The American Journal of Preventive Medicine* 10: 77–84. [CrossRef]

Arora, Teresa, and Ian Grey. 2020. Health behaviour changes during COVID-19 and the potential consequences: A mini-review. *Journal of Health Psychology* 25: 1155–63. [CrossRef]

Balkhi, Fizra, Aamna Nasir, Arhama Zehra, and Ramsha Riaz. 2020. Psychological and behavioral response to the coronavirus (COVID-19) pandemic. *Cureus* 12: e7923. [CrossRef]

Caputo, Eduardo L., and Felipe F. Reichert. 2020. Studies of physical activity and COVID-19 during the pandemic: A scoping review. *Journal of Physical Activity and Health* 17: 1275–84. [CrossRef] [PubMed]

Cheng, Cindy, Joan Barceló, Allison Spencer Hartnett, Robert Kubinec, and Luca Messerschmidt. 2020. COVID-19 government response event dataset (CoronaNet v. 1.0). *Nature Human Behaviour* 4: 756–68. [CrossRef]

Codagnone, Cristiano, Francesco Bogliacino, Camilo Gómez, Rafael Charris, Felipe Montealegre, Giovanni Liva, Francisco Lupiáñez-Villanueva, Frans Folkvord, and Giuseppe A. Veltri. 2020. Assessing concerns for the economic consequence of the COVID-19 response and mental health problems associated with economic vulnerability and negative economic shock in Italy, Spain, and the United Kingdom. *PLoS ONE* 15: e0240876. [CrossRef]

Center for Systems Science and Engineering (CSSE) at Johns Hopkins University, USA. 2021. Available online: https://gisanddata.maps.arcgis.com/apps/opsdashboard/index.html#/bda7594740fd40299423467b48e9ecf6 (accessed on 26 September 2021).

Cunningham, Conor, Roger O'Sullivan, Paolo Caserotti, and Mark A. Tully. 2020. Consequences of physical inactivity in older adults: A systematic review of reviews and meta-analyses. *The Scandinavian Journal of Medicine & Science in Sports* 30: 816–27. [CrossRef]

De Jong Gierveld, Jenny, and Theo Van Tilburg. 1999. Manual of the loneliness scale 1999. Department of Social Research Methodology, Vrije Universiteit Amsterdam, Amsterdam (Updated Version 1801 02). Available online: https://home.fsw.vu.nl/TG.van.Tilburg/manual_loneliness_scale_1999.html (accessed on 26 September 2021).

Duan, Yanping, Sonia Lippke, Wei Liang, Borui Shang, Wagner Petra, Julien Steven Baker, Jiali He, and Franziska Marie Keller. 2021. Association of social-cognitive factors with individual preventive behaviors of Covid-19 among a mixed-sample of older adults from China and Germany. *Res-Square*. Available online: https://www.researchsquare.com/article/rs-503762/v1 (accessed on 26 September 2021). [CrossRef]

Dwyer, Michael John, Margherita Pasini, Stefano De Dominicis, and Elda Righi. 2020. Physical activity: Benefits and challenges during the COVID-19 pandemic. *The Scandinavian Journal of Medicine & Science in Sports* 30: 1291. [CrossRef]

Gehlich, Kerstin H., Johannes Beller, Bernhard Lange-Asschenfeldt, Wolfgang Köcher, Martina C. Meinke, and Jürgen Lademann. 2019. Fruit and vegetable consumption is associated with improved mental and cognitive health in older adults from non-Western developing countries. *Public Health Nutrition* 22: 689–96. [CrossRef] [PubMed]

Hu, Zhao, Xuhui Lin, Atipatsa Chiwanda Kaminga, and Huilan Xu. 2020. Impact of the COVID-19 epidemic on lifestyle behaviors and their association with subjective well-being among the general population in mainland China: Cross-sectional study. *The Journal of Medical Internet Research* 22: e21176. [CrossRef]

Hu, Xinyi, Antoine Flahault, Alexander Temerev, and Liudmila Rozanova. 2021. The Progression of COVID-19 and the Government Response in China. *International Journal of Environmental Research and Public Health* 18: 3002. [CrossRef] [PubMed]

Jin, Huajie, Haiyin Wang, Xiao Li, Weiwei Zheng, Shanke Ye, Sheng Zhang, Jiahui Zhou, and Mark Pennington. 2021. Economic burden of COVID-19, China, January–March, 2020: A cost-of-illness study. *Bulletin of the World Health Organization* 99: 112. [CrossRef]

Khan, Kiran Shafiq, Mohammed A. Mamun, Mark D. Griffiths, and Irfan Ullah. 2020. The mental health impact of the COVID-19 pandemic across different cohorts. *International Journal of Mental Health and Addiction* 9: 1–7. [CrossRef]

Kingsbury, Mila, Gabrielle Dupuis, Felice Jacka, Marie-Hélène Roy-Gagnon, Seanna E. McMartin, and Ian Colman. 2016. Associations between fruit and vegetable consumption and depressive symptoms: Evidence from a national Canadian longitudinal survey. *Journal of Epidemiology and Community Health* 70: 155–61. [CrossRef] [PubMed]

Leung, Grace Tak Yu, Jenny de Jong Gierveld, and Linda Chiu Wa Lam. 2008. Validation of the Chinese translation of the 6-item De Jong Gierveld Loneliness Scale in elderly Chinese. *International Psychogeriatrics* 20: 1262–72. [CrossRef]

Li, Xiaojing, and Qinliang Liu. 2020. Social media use, eHealth literacy, disease knowledge, and preventive behaviors in the COVID-19 pandemic: Cross-sectional study on Chinese netizens. *Journal of Medical Internet Research* 22: e19684. [CrossRef]

Li, Siyue, Bo Feng, Wang Liao, and Wenjing Pan. 2020. Internet use, risk awareness, and demographic characteristics associated with engagement in preventive behaviors and testing: Cross-sectional survey on COVID-19 in the United States. *The Journal of Medical Internet Research* 22: e19782. [CrossRef] [PubMed]

Liang, Wei, Yan Ping Duan, Bo Rui Shang, Yan Ping Wang, Chun Hu, and Sonia Lippke. 2019. A web-based lifestyle intervention program for Chinese college students: Study protocol and baseline characteristics of a randomized placebo-controlled trial. *BMC Public Health* 19: 1. [CrossRef]

Liang, Wei, Yanping Duan, Borui Shang, Chun Hu, Julien Steven Baker, Zhihua Lin, Jiali He, and Yanping Wang. 2021. Precautionary behavior and depression in older adults during the COVID-19 pandemic: An online cross-sectional study in Hubei, China. *International Journal of Environmental Research and Public Health* 18: 1853. [CrossRef]

Litton, Michelle M., and Alyssa W. Beavers. 2020. The Relationship between Food Security Status and Fruit and Vegetable Intake during the COVID-19 Pandemic. *Nutrients* 13: 712. [CrossRef] [PubMed]

Liu, Hua-Xuan, Bik-Chu Chow, Wei Liang, Holger Hassel, and YaJun Wendy Huang. 2021. Measuring a broad spectrum of eHealth skills in the Web 3.0 context using an eHealth Literacy Scale: Development and validation study. *The Journal of Medical Internet Research* 23: e31627. [CrossRef]

López-Bueno, Rubén, Guillermo F. López-Sánchez, José A. Casajús, Joaquín Calatayud, Alejandro Gil-Salmerón, Igor Grabovac, Mark A. Tully, and Lee Smith. 2020. Health-related behaviors among school-aged children and adolescents during the Spanish Covid-19 confinement. *Frontiers in Pediatrics* 8: 573. [CrossRef] [PubMed]

National Health Commission of China. 2021. Update on the New Coronavirus Cases. Available online: http://health.people.com.cn/GB/26466/431463/431576/index.html (accessed on 26 September 2021).

Pels, Fabian, and Jens Kleinert. 2016. Loneliness and physical activity: A systematic review. *International Review of Sport and Exercise Psychology* 9: 231–60. [CrossRef]

Pinquart, Martin. 2001. Correlates of subjective health in older adults: A meta-analysis. *Psychology and Aging* 16: 414. [CrossRef] [PubMed]

Probst, Tahira M., Hyun Jung Lee, and Andrea Bazzoli. 2020. Economic stressors and the enactment of CDC-recommended COVID-19 prevention behaviors: The impact of state-level context. *The Journal of Applied Psychology* 105: 1397–407. [CrossRef]

Puspitasari, Irma Melyani, Lutfiah Yusuf, Rano K. Sinuraya, Rizky Abdulah, and Hiroshi Koyama. 2020. Knowledge, attitude, and practice during the COVID-19 pandemic: A review. *The Journal of Multidisciplinary Healthcare* 13: 727. [CrossRef]

Qin, Fei, Yiqing Song, George P. Nassis, Lina Zhao, Yanan Dong, Cuicui Zhao, Yiwei Feng, and Jiexiu Zhao. 2020. Physical activity, screen time, and emotional well-being during the 2019 novel coronavirus outbreak in China. *International Journal of Environmental Research and Public Health* 17: 5170. [CrossRef]

Rankin, Sally H., Michael E. Galbraith, and Sharon Johnson. 1993. Reliability and validity data for a Chinese translation of the Center for Epidemiological Studies-Depression. *Psychological Reports* 73: 1291–98. [CrossRef]

Schrack, Jennifer A., Amal A. Wanigatunga, and Stephen P. Juraschek. 2020. After the COVID-19 pandemic: The next wave of health challenges for older adults. *The Journals of Gerontology* 75: e121–2. [CrossRef] [PubMed]

Selya, Arielle S., Jennifer S. Rose, Lisa C. Dierker, Donald Hedeker, and Robin J. Mermelstein. 2012. A practical guide to calculating Cohen's f2, a measure of local effect size, from PROC MIXED. *Frontiers in Psychology* 3: 111. [CrossRef]

Shahid, Zainab, Ricci Kalayanamitra, Brendan McClafferty, Douglas Kepko, Devyani Ramgobin, Ravi Patel, Chander Shekher Aggarwal, Ramarao Vunnam, Nitasa Sahu, Dhirisha Bhatt, and et al. 2020. COVID-19 and older adults: What we know. *Journal of the American Geriatrics Society* 68: 926–29. [CrossRef]

Shankar, Aparna, Anne McMunn, and Andrew Steptoe. 2010. Health-related behaviors in older adults: Relationships with socioeconomic status. *The American Journal of Preventive Medicine* 38: 39–46. [CrossRef]

Singh, Jaspreet, and Jagandeep Singh. 2020. COVID-19 and its impact on society. *Electronic Research Journal of Social Sciences and Humanities* 2. Available online: https://ssrn.com/abstract=3567837 (accessed on 26 September 2021).

Stickley, Andrew, Tetsuya Matsubayashi, Hajime Sueki, and Michiko Ueda. 2020. COVID-19 preventive behaviours among people with anxiety and depressive symptoms: Findings from Japan. *Public Health* 189: 91–3. [CrossRef]

Usher, Kim, Debra Jackson, Joanne Durkin, Naomi Gyamfi, and Navjot Bhullar. 2020. Pandemic-related behaviours and psychological outcomes; A rapid literature review to explain COVID-19 behaviours. *International Journal of Mental Health Nursing* 29: 1018–34. [CrossRef]

Vahia, Ipsit V., Dilip V. Jeste, and Charles F. Reynolds. 2020. Older adults and the mental health effects of COVID-19. *JAMA* 324: 2253–4. [CrossRef]

Wang, Cuiyan, Riyu Pan, Xiaoyang Wan, Yilin Tan, Linkang Xu, Cyrus S. Ho, and Roger C. Ho. 2020. Immediate psychological responses and associated factors during the initial stage of the 2019 coronavirus disease (COVID-19) epidemic among the general population in China. *International Journal of Environmental Research and Public Health* 17: 1729. [CrossRef]

Wang, Cuiyan, Riyu Pan, Xiaoyang Wan, Yilin Tan, Linkang Xu, Roger S. McIntyre, Faith N. Choo, B. Tran, R. Ho, Vijay K. Sharma, and et al. 2020. A longitudinal study on the mental health of general population during the COVID-19 epidemic in China. *Brain, Behavior, and Immunity* 87: 40–48. [CrossRef] [PubMed]

Weaver, Raven H., Alexandra Jackson, Jane Lanigan, Thomas G. Power, Alana Anderson, Anne E. Cox, Linda Eddy, Louise Parker, Yoshie Sano, and Elizabeth Weybright. 2021. Health Behaviors at the Onset of the COVID-19 Pandemic. *The American Journal of Health Behavior* 45: 44–61. [CrossRef] [PubMed]

World Health Organization. 2020. Coronavirus Disease (COVID-19) Pandemic. Available online: https://www.who.int/emergencies/diseases/novel-coronavirus-2019 (accessed on 15 October 2020).

WHO. 2021a. WHO Coronavirus Disease (COVID-19) Dashboard. Available online: https://covid19.who.int/ (accessed on 26 September 2021).
WHO. 2021b. World Health Organization. Coronavirus Disease (COVID-19) Advice for the Public. Available online: https://www.who.int/emergencies/diseases/novel-coronavirus-2019/advice-for-public (accessed on 30 August 2021).
Wilczyńska, Dominika, Jianye Li, Yin Yang, Hongying Fan, Taofeng Liu, and Mariusz Lipowski. 2021. Fear of COVID-19 changes the motivation for physical activity participation: Polish-Chinese comparisons. *Health Psychology Report* 2: 138–48. Available online: https://czasopisma.bg.ug.edu.pl/index.php/HPR/article/view/5754 (accessed on 26 September 2021).
Wu, Bei. 2020. Social isolation and loneliness among older adults in the context of COVID-19: A global challenge. *Global Health Res and Policy* 5: 1–3. [CrossRef] [PubMed]
Yahia, Elhadi M., María Elena Maldonado Celis, and Mette Svendsen. 2017. The contribution of fruit and vegetable consumption to human health. In *Fruit and vegetable Phytochemicals*. Edited by E. M. Yahia. Hoboken: John Wiley & Sons, vol. 29, pp. 3–52.
Yang, Yuan, Wen Li, Qinge Zhang, Ling Zhang, Teris Cheung, and Yu-Tao Xiang. 2020. Mental health services for older adults in China during the COVID-19 outbreak. *The Lancet Psychiatry* 7: e19. [CrossRef]
Ye, Yisheng, Ruoxi Wang, Da Feng, Ruijun Wu, Zhifei Li, Chengxu Long, Zhanchun Feng, and Shangfeng Tang. 2020. The recommended and excessive preventive behaviors during the COVID-19 pandemic: A community-based online survey in China. *International Journal of Environmental Research and Public Health* 17: 6953. [CrossRef]

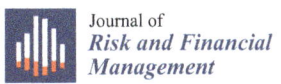

Editorial

Financial Burden and Shortage of Respiratory Rehabilitation for SARS-CoV-2 Survivors: The Next Step of the Pandemic?

Frédéric Dutheil [1,2], Maelys Clinchamps [2], Julien S. Baker [3], Rashmi Supriya [3,*], Alistair Cole [4], Yang Gao [3] and Valentin Navel [5,6]

[1] CNRS, LaPSCo, Physiological and Psychosocial Stress, University Clermont Auvergne, F-63000 Clermont-Ferrand, France; frederic.dutheil@uca.fr
[2] Preventive and Occupational Medicine, University Hospital of Clermont-Ferrand, F-63000 Clermont-Ferrand, France; maelysclinchamps@gmail.com
[3] Centre for Health and Exercise Science Research, Department of Sport, Physical Education and Health, Hong Kong Baptist University, Kowloon Tong, Hong Kong 999077, China; jsbaker@hkbu.edu.hk (J.S.B.); gaoyang@hkbu.edu.hk (Y.G.)
[4] Department of Government and International Studies, Hong Kong Baptist University, Kowloon Tong, Hong Kong 999077, China; alistaircole@hkbu.edu.hk
[5] CNRS, INSERM, GReD, Translational Approach to Epithelial Injury and Repair, University Clermont Auvergne, F-63000 Clermont-Ferrand, France; valentin.navel@hotmail.fr
[6] Ophthalmology, University Hospital of Clermont-Ferrand, CHU Clermont-Ferrand, F-63000 Clermont-Ferrand, France
* Correspondence: Rashmisupriya@hkbu.edu.hk

Citation: Dutheil, Frédéric, Maelys Clinchamps, Julien S. Baker, Rashmi Supriya, Alistair Cole, Yang Gao, and Valentin Navel. 2022. Financial Burden and Shortage of Respiratory Rehabilitation for SARS-CoV-2 Survivors: The Next Step of the Pandemic? *Journal of Risk and Financial Management* 15: 20. https://doi.org/10.3390/jrfm15010020

Received: 30 November 2021
Accepted: 29 December 2021
Published: 7 January 2022

Publisher's Note: MDPI stays neutral with regard to jurisdictional claims in published maps and institutional affiliations.

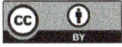

Copyright: © 2022 by the authors. Licensee MDPI, Basel, Switzerland. This article is an open access article distributed under the terms and conditions of the Creative Commons Attribution (CC BY) license (https://creativecommons.org/licenses/by/4.0/).

We read with great enthusiasm the recent article by Daynes et al. highlighting the encouraging outcomes of COVID-19 rehabilitation (Daynes et al. 2021). Indeed, results for exercise capacity, health related quality of life, anxiety, and depression seemed to improve following 6 weeks of rehabilitation. In chronic respiratory diseases, such as chronic obstructive pulmonary disease (COPD), respiratory rehabilitation (RR) has demonstrated benefits both in terms of respiratory symptoms (Ward et al. 2020) and mental health (Gordon et al. 2019). RR centers are the cornerstone of patient management (Ward et al. 2020). In spite of the known benefits of RR, in reality, patients are not as likely to attend, and complete RR as required. Transportation, hospital capacities, and staffing issues are often overlooked as impediment factors in RR compliance. In fact, some studies have shown that the most common barrier to participation in RR is insufficient transportation to and from hospital-based programs (Wadell et al. 2013; Thorpe et al. 2012). In 2015, the official ATS/ERS Policy Statement on Enhancing Implementation noted that further barriers to RR were highlighted in the delivery of RR (Rochester et al. 2015). Health professionals, payers, patients, and caregivers lack awareness and knowledge of the benefits of RR; the optimal use of RR by suitable patient populations (Jones et al. 2014); and limited training opportunities for RR providers. The use of telerehabilitation is another potential method to overcome the limitations of traditional hospital-based RR (Salawu et al. 2020; Sivan et al. 2020). Using information and communication technologies to provide clinical rehabilitation services over the internet has been classified as telerehabilitation (Kairy et al. 2009). In 2021, it was reported that during the treatment of chronic COPD, the need for continuous treatment and care, and the high costs of medications and RR services led to a heavy financial burden for patients and their families. In contrast, the stress and concern caused by the inability to receive medication and to participate in RR worsened the condition. As a result, RR is often not continued by patients and their families (Sami et al. 2021). A Canadian Economic Analysis, published in 2010, showed that normal care plus RR is 27% more effective than usual care, with incremental cost-effectiveness ratios of Canadian dollar (CAD) 27,924 per additional quality-adjusted life-year gained. The authors also reported that, over a 10-year period, if COPD patients were only treated in moderate and severe cases, then 1505 additional people would receive RR treatment in Canada at an added cost of CAD 1.8 million per year. In the case of a 25% increase in COPD patients needing RR, the cost would rise to CAD 33.9 million. The additional annual cost for all individuals with COPD (100% treatment) who require RR would be CAD 168 million (CADTH 2010).

The novel Coronavirus-19 (COVID-19) pandemic mainly affects the respiratory tract. Older adults with comorbid conditions are particularly vulnerable. Post-intensive care syndrome (PICS) is more likely to develop in patients weaned from mechanical ventilation. COVID-19 is an infectious disease responsible for several symptoms, such as fever, tiredness, dry cough, difficulty breathing, pneumonia, and respiratory failure (Velavan and Meyer 2020). Even if the most infected patients recover from the disease without specialist treatment, the remaining population, especially those with underlying comorbidities, tend to develop difficulty in breathing. This condition progresses from mild to severe, and eventually results in critical case diagnosis. Generally, critical cases who develop an acute respiratory distress syndrome (ARDS) are sent to intensive care units (ICU). Because of the severity of lung damage and because of the common phylogenetic association with coronaviruses, COVID-19 was renamed severe acute respiratory syndrome coronavirus 2 (SARS-CoV-2) (Jiang et al. 2020). In the worst-case scenario, patients evolve towards respiratory failure due to lung deterioration, and if they survive, can cause long-term lung failure (Xu et al. 2020). The major sequelae caused by the virus increase the need for respiratory rehabilitation for SARS-Cov-2 survivors. Moreover, even patients from the general population who did not require an ICU stay may also need respiratory rehabilitation. This results from the fact that more than half of the patients with pneumonia presented with bilateral multifocal lung lesions, such as ground glass and linear opacities, adjacent pleura, or interlobular thickening (Xu et al. 2020). Although not evaluated, some suggestions of home respiratory rehabilitation programs for patients in quarantine have been proposed, with the use of connected and developed technologies for rehabilitation guidance (Zhao et al. 2020).

All aspects of health care delivery have been greatly affected by the COVID-19 pandemic. A number of changes have been implemented to rules, regulations, and reimbursement policies in order to protect health care workers and patients from the transmission of the disease (Centers for Medicare and Medicaid Services 2020). Numerous organizations have expanded their resources and advice for the implementation of telerehabilitation services as a reaction to this new landscape of medical practice, including the American Physical Therapy Association, Australian Physiotherapy Association, and Italian Physiotherapy Association. Physical therapy services were deemed essential by federal, state, and local authorities during the pandemic, as reported in the Report from the American Physical Therapy Association published in June 2020 (American Physiotherapy Association 2020). Yet, many physical therapists have actively curtailed their hours to "flatten the curve" of the pandemic by reducing patient contact time. In the midst of a pandemic, the American Physical Therapy Association recommends video conferencing to allow physical therapists to communicate directly with clients. Since patients with COPD are especially susceptible to severe COVID-19 complications, in-person RR should not take place during the pandemic except in exceptional cases (Lippi and Henry 2020; Zhao et al. 2020). It may be possible to conduct in-person RR only when COVID-19 has a low community spread. It is recommended to wear acceptable personal protective equipment (PPE) at all times for those physical trainers who will have to provide care in person during the pandemic. Numerous respondents commented that their PPE supplies were inadequate despite these recommendations.

Mobile health technologies have demonstrated some positive possibilities for respiratory disease rehabilitation (MacKinnon and Brittain 2020), and the technologies proposed might be useful as a support mechanism for survivors of SARS-CoV-2. Due to telerehabilitation's high cost, it is important to make sure that it is implemented according to sound clinical policy decisions and high-quality evidence. Telerehabilitation holds great potential as a "therapeutic" tool for a large number of COPD patients during and after the COVID-19 pandemic, if these challenges can be overcome (Burkow et al. 2015). Telerehabilitation is underfunded in most jurisdictions. These programs need funding in order to develop a solid foundation of evidence for their use and to sustain the treatment in the community. In the past, most insurers around the world would reimburse PR for outpatient rehabilitation but not telerehabilitation prior to the COVID pandemic (Garvey et al. 2018; Bierman et al. 2018). The uptake of telerehabilitation in US health care systems has been constrained by variations and restrictions in state regulations and reimbursement policies of private and Medicare insurers, according to a 2018 report by Bierman et al. 2018. Telerehabilitation could be used in the community more often if funding was provided for the technology. However, these technological developments would not provide sufficient medical benefits for the most severe SARS-CoV-2 patients who have been subjected to mechanical ventilation in ICU. Even if recommendations exist for respiratory physiotherapy for patients hospitalized in ICU with invasive mechanical ventilation (Lazzeri et al. 2020), there is still no consensus or guidelines on the best rehabilitation procedures for survivors following treatment in ICU. As more patients recover from COVID-19 and are stable enough to enter post-acute rehabilitation care, nursing homes are declining to admit these patients because of their inability to provide efficient care in a safe environment. Due to decreased Medicare revenues and increased costs related to managing patients with COVID-19, some nursing homes are facing bankruptcy (Grabowski and Mor 2020). There is an urgent need for the rehabilitation of survivors in specialized centers; however, specialized rehabilitation establishments already lack reception capacities and have long waiting lists.

Moreover, rehabilitation medicine has a holistic dimension that is essential for SARS-Cov-2 survivors who may have problems with sarcopenia, usually as a consequence of hospitalization in ICU (Gropper et al. 2019). Sarcopenia development in SARS-Cov-2 survivors may be of multifactorial origin and could include neuromyopathy, muscular dysfunction linked to respiratory failure, neurological damage specific to the virus (neurotropism), cardiovascular disorders (endothelitis), undernutrition, or common frequent comorbidities recorded in the most vulnerable SARS-CoV-2 elderly patients (e.g., obesity, diabetes) (Cruz-Jentoft and Sayer 2019). Finally, the overall functional dimension of physical and rehabilitation medicine is useful for SARS-CoV-2 survivors. Despite global efforts to limit the spread of the SARS-CoV-2, we draw attention towards the need to plan for optimal respiratory and general rehabilitation of SARS-CoV-2 survivors. The next major problem related to infection rate of the pandemic might be a shortage of respiratory rehabilitation centers, which may also collaterally affect patients with other chronic respiratory diseases. In response to the COVID-19 pandemic, RR has undergone dramatic changes. Some of these changes are practical venue changes and increased use of telerehabilitation. In addition to revealing longstanding structural barriers to RR, the pandemic has highlighted the lack of funding, resources, and healthcare professionals, which have been exacerbated by COVID-19. This has been compromised further by the economic burden of the pandemic, shortages of healthcare staff and equipment, and diminished hospital and healthcare facilities.

Author Contributions: F.D., M.C., V.N., J.S.B. and R.S. wrote the paper. A.C. and Y.G. contributed to discussion and editing. All authors have read and agreed to the published version of the manuscript.

Funding: This research received no external funding.

Institutional Review Board Statement: Not applicable.

Informed Consent Statement: Not applicable.

Data Availability Statement: Not applicable.

Acknowledgments: This paper was prepared from the presentation on idea presented in the symposium "Transnational and Transdisciplinary Lessons of COVID-19 From the Perspective of Risk and Management".

Conflicts of Interest: The authors declare no conflict of interest.

References

American Physiotherapy Association. 2020. Impact of COVID-19 on the Physical Therapy Profession: A Report from the American Physical Therapy Association. Available online: https://www.naranet.org/uploads/userfiles/files/documents/APTAReportImpactOfCOVID-19OnThePhysicalTherapyProfession.pdf (accessed on 29 July 2021).

Bierman, Randal Trey, Mei Wa Kwong, and Christine Calouro. 2018. State Occupational and Physical Therapy Telehealth Laws and Regulations: A 50-State Survey. *International Journal of Telerehabilitation* 10: 3–54. [CrossRef] [PubMed]

Burkow, Tatjana M., Lars K. Vognild, Elin Johnsen, Marijke Jongsma Risberg, Astrid Bratvold, Elin Breivik, Trine Krogstad, and Audhild Hjalmarsen. 2015. Comprehensive pulmonary rehabilitation in home-based online groups: A mixed method pilot study in COPD. *BMC Research Notes* 8: 766. [CrossRef]

CADTH. 2010. Pulmonary rehabilitation for chronic obstructive pulmonary disease: Clinical, economic, and budget impact analysis. *CADTH Technology Overviews* 1: e0127. Available online: http://www.ncbi.nlm.nih.gov/pubmed/22977417 (accessed on 29 July 2021).

Centers for Medicare and Medicaid Services. 2020. COVID-19 Emergency Declaration Blanket Waivers for Health Care Providers. Available online: https://www.cms.gov/files/document/summary-covid-19-emergency-declaration-waivers.pdf (accessed on 2 August 2021).

Cruz-Jentoft, Alfonso J., and Avan A. Sayer. 2019. Sarcopenia. *The Lancet* 393: 2636–46. [CrossRef]

Daynes, Enya, Charlotte Gerlis, Emma Chaplin, Nikki Gardiner, and Sally J. Singh. 2021. Early experiences of rehabilitation for individuals post-COVID to improve fatigue, breathlessness exercise capacity and cognition—A cohort study. *Chronic Respiratory Disease* 18: 147997312110156. [CrossRef]

Garvey, Chris, Jonathan P. Singer, Allan Murphy Bruun, Allison Soong, Julia Rigler, and Steven Hays. 2018. Moving Pulmonary Rehabilitation Into the Home. *Journal of Cardiopulmonary Rehabilitation and Prevention* 38: 8–16. [CrossRef] [PubMed]

Gordon, Carla S., Jacob W. Waller, Rylee M. Cook, Steffan L. Cavalera, Wing T. Lim, and Christian R. Osadnik. 2019. Effect of Pulmonary Rehabilitation on Symptoms of Anxiety and Depression in COPD. *Chest* 156: 80–91. [CrossRef] [PubMed]

Grabowski, David C., and Vincent Mor. 2020. Nursing Home Care in Crisis in the Wake of COVID-19. *JAMA* 324: 23. [CrossRef]

Gropper, Sareen, Dennis Hunt, and Deborah W. Chapa. 2019. Sarcopenia and Psychosocial Variables in Patients in Intensive Care Units. *Critical Care Nursing Clinics of North America* 31: 489–99. [CrossRef]

Jiang, Shibo, Zhengli Shi, Yuelong Shu, Jingdong Song, George F. Gao, Wenjie Tan, and Deyin Guo. 2020. A distinct name is needed for the new coronavirus. *The Lancet* 395: 949. [CrossRef]

Jones, Sarah E., Stuart A. Green, Amy L. Clark, Mandy J. Dickson, Ann-Marie Nolan, Clare Moloney, Samantha S. C. Kon, Faisal Kamal, Joy Godden, Cathy Howe, and et al. 2014. Pulmonary rehabilitation following hospitalisation for acute exacerbation of COPD: Referrals, uptake and adherence. *Thorax* 69: 181–82. [CrossRef] [PubMed]

Kairy, Dahlia, Pascale Lehoux, Claude Vincent, and Martha Visintin. 2009. A systematic review of clinical outcomes, clinical process, healthcare utilization and costs associated with telerehabilitation. *Disability and Rehabilitation* 31: 427–47. [CrossRef]

Lazzeri, Marta, Andrea Lanza, Raffaella Bellini, Angela Bellofiore, Simone Cecchetto, Alessia Colombo, Francesco D'Abrosca, Cesare Del Monaco, Giuseppe Gaudiello, Mara Paneroni, and et al. 2020. Respiratory physiotherapy in patients with COVID-19 infection in acute setting: A Position Paper of the Italian Association of Respiratory Physiotherapists (ARIR). *Monaldi Archives for Chest Disease* 90. [CrossRef]

Lippi, Giuseppe, and Brandon Michael Henry. 2020. Chronic obstructive pulmonary disease is associated with severe coronavirus disease 2019 (COVID-19). *Respiratory Medicine* 167: 105941. [CrossRef]

MacKinnon, Grant E., and Evan L. Brittain. 2020. Mobile Health Technologies in Cardiopulmonary Disease. *Chest* 157: 654–64. [CrossRef] [PubMed]

Rochester, Carolyn L., Ioannis Vogiatzis, Anne E. Holland, Suzanne C. Lareau, Darcy D. Marciniuk, Milo A. Puhan, Martijn A. Spruit, Sarah Masefield, Richard Casaburi, Enrico M. Clini, and et al. 2015. An Official American Thoracic Society/European Respiratory Society Policy Statement: Enhancing Implementation, Use, and Delivery of Pulmonary Rehabilitation. *American Journal of Respiratory and Critical Care Medicine* 192: 1373–86. [CrossRef]

Salawu, Abayomi, Angela Green, Michael G. Crooks, Nina Brixey, Denise H. Ross, and Manoj Sivan. 2020. A Proposal for Multidisciplinary Tele-Rehabilitation in the Assessment and Rehabilitation of COVID-19 Survivors. *International Journal of Environmental Research and Public Health* 17: 4890. [CrossRef]

Sami, Ramin, Kobra Salehi, Marzieh Hashemi, and Vajihe Atashi. 2021. Exploring the barriers to pulmonary rehabilitation for patients with chronic obstructive pulmonary disease: A qualitative study. *BMC Health Services Research* 21: 828. [CrossRef] [PubMed]

Sivan, Manoj, Stephen Halpin, Lisa Hollingworth, Niki Snook, Katherine Hickman, and Ian J. Clifton. 2020. Development of an integrated rehabilitation pathway for individuals recovering from COVID-19 in the community. *Journal of Rehabilitation Medicine* 52. [CrossRef]

Thorpe, Olivia, Kylie Johnston, and Saravana Kumar. 2012. Barriers and Enablers to Physical Activity Participation in Patients With COPD. *Journal of Cardiopulmonary Rehabilitation and Prevention* 32: 359–69. [CrossRef]

Velavan, Thirumalaisamy P., and Christian G. Meyer. 2020. The COVID-19 epidemic. *Tropical Medicine & International Health* 25: 278–80. [CrossRef]

Wadell, Karin, T. Janaudis Ferreira, Mats Arne, Karin Lisspers, Björn Ställberg, and Margareta Emtner. 2013. Hospital-based pulmonary rehabilitation in patients with COPD in Sweden–A national survey. *Respiratory Medicine* 107: 1195–200. [CrossRef]

Ward, Thomas JC, Charles D. Plumptre, Thomas E. Dolmage, Amy V. Jones, Ruth Trethewey, Pip Divall, Sally J. Singh, Martin R. Lindley, Michael C. Steiner, and Rachael A. Evans. 2020. Change in O2peak in Response to Aerobic Exercise Training and the Relationship With Exercise Prescription in People With COPD: A Systematic Review and Meta-analysis. *Chest* 158: 131–44. [CrossRef] [PubMed]

Xu, Xi, Chengcheng Yu, Jing Qu, Lieguang Zhang, Songfeng Jiang, Deyang Huang, Bihua Chen, Zhiping Zhang, Wanhua Guan, Zhoukun Ling, and et al. 2020. Imaging and clinical features of patients with 2019 novel coronavirus SARS-CoV-2. *European Journal of Nuclear Medicine and Molecular Imaging* 47: 1275–80. [CrossRef]

Zhao, Hong-Mei, Yu-Xiao Xie, and Chen Wang. 2020. Recommendations for respiratory rehabilitation in adults with coronavirus disease 2019. *Chinese Medical Journal* 133: 1595–602. [CrossRef] [PubMed]

Zhao, Qianwen, Meng Meng, Rahul Kumar, Yinlian Wu, Jiaofeng Huang, Ningfang Lian, Yunlei Deng, and Su Lin. 2020. The impact of COPD and smoking history on the severity of COVID-19: A systemic review and meta-analysis. *Journal of Medical Virology* 92: 1915–21. [CrossRef] [PubMed]

Editorial

Alcohol Consumption Pre and Post COVID-19. Implications for Health, Underlying Pathologies, Risks and Its Management

Julien S. Baker, Rashmi Supriya *, Dan Tao and Yang Gao

Centre for Health and Exercise Science Research, Department of Sport, Physical Education and Health, Hong Kong Baptist University, Kowloon Tong 999077, Hong Kong; jsbaker@hkbu.edu.hk (J.S.B.); emma0514@hkbu.edu.hk (D.T.); gaoyang@hkbu.edu.hk (Y.G.)
* Correspondence: Rashmisupriya@hkbu.edu.hk

Research indicates that individuals who experience increased levels of stress often report increased alcohol consumption and consequently misuse. Individuals who have experiences related to financial problems or anxiety and depressive issues often rely on alcohol consumption as a short-term solution for symptom relief. However, this strategy often results in an increase in the severity of alcohol misuse, addiction and dependence. In support of this, previous research has revealed that sections of a Chinese population who were isolated working in quiet locations during the 2003 SARS epidemic used alcohol to deal with isolation, and perceived increases in stress. The increase in alcohol consumption during this period was significantly related to incidences of alcohol abuse and dependence several years post the SARS epidemic (Grossman et al. 2020). The continued increase in the COVID-19 pandemic and government measures to impose isolation, travel restrictions mobility limitations, and decreased socialization have had a powerful impact on individuals' patterns of leisure time. This has also resulted in a decrease in individual access to venues that publicly sell alcohol. This has had implications for increased alcohol consumption in the home environment. Recovery from the impact of the pandemic will remain for long periods. The recovery periods during and following the pandemic may increase the potential for individual engagement in alcohol consumption and misuse to alleviate the continuing problems associated with isolation, anxiety and depression caused by COVID-19 (Hou et al. 2021).

Research has also outlined that during the COVID-19 pandemic, in addition to the increased stress levels recorded, domestic violence increased and was associated with excessive alcohol consumption as a contributory factor (Gama et al. 2020). Alcohol abuse can contribute to individual health profiles, impact negatively on diseases, promote personal injury, and make abusers more susceptible to the physiological and psychological effects of COVID-19. In addition, alcohol abuse can also lead to significant economic and social problems (Moss 2013). During the pandemic, a large proportion of the population did not increase their alcohol consumption. However, for the individuals who did increase consumption, a greater proportion appeared to consume larger quantities. In the USA, alcohol sales increased exponentially by 234%. Quarantine and social isolation have had a huge psychological effect on people's lives, and these effects may be responsible for the increase in alcohol misuse observed in adults (Pollard et al. 2020). Figures from the World Health Organization have indicated that alcohol misuse accounts for more than 5% of global diseases (WHO 2018). In relation to the COVID-19 pandemic, individuals that abuse alcohol or have underlying medical pathologies such as alcohol-related diseased livers and associated comorbidities are at an increased risk of serious illness or premature death.

Societal impacts of long-term lockdowns and associated isolation stressors during the pandemic contribute to these problems in compromised individuals and have huge implications and relevance for issues related to public health (Clay and Parker 2020). Rehm et al. (2020) suggested that there are two different scenarios related to how the

COVID-19 pandemic may affect alcohol consumers. The first scenario, in an attempt to limit alcohol consumption, includes limits on alcohol availability, financial constraints on alcohol purchases, and governmental limitations that would help reduce the levels of alcohol consumed. The second scenario relates to the negative effects of increased stress and anxiety for individuals who resort to alcohol misuse to alleviate pandemic effects. Alcohol abuse is a very serious and increasing public health concern. There are about 65,000 US deaths with approximately 4% of fatalities and 5% of diseases and associated injuries worldwide that can be attributed directly to alcohol abuse (NIAAA 2021). Drinking populations can be categorized into sub sections. These sections include drinkers with severe alcohol misuse problems and individuals who exceed recommended guidelines but fail to reach the severity of severe alcohol misuse. For example, in America 25% of adults and somewhere between 7% and 20% of adult primary care patients exceed recommended drinking guidelines (NIAAA 2021). Excessive alcohol abuse is related to an increase in the prevalence of several serious medical conditions. These include but are not limited to certain cancers, cardiovascular disease, the related comorbidities of cirrhosis and pancreatitis, and gastrointestinal disorders. In addition to this, excessive alcohol misuse has also been associated with an increased risk of gastrointestinal related hospitalizations, postoperative complications, and poorer self-management of chronic diseases, such as diabetes, and hypertension. A study by Kuitunen-Paul and Roerecke (2018) reported that even consuming alcohol at moderate levels can increase all-cause mortality and contribute to the risk of cardiovascular related diseases while reducing life expectancy.

Further guidelines have reported that excessive alcohol consumption results in increased blood pressure and risks of stroke. The guidelines suggest that even moderate drinking (two drinks per day or less) increase the risk of stroke by about 15% (NIAAA 2021). While there is evidence for problems associated with alcohol abuse and misuse, there is little research assessing the effects of alcohol consumption on individuals with underlying medical conditions. The consumption of alcohol, particularly drinking large amounts, is a contributory factor for many alcohol related health issues. Alcohol consumption is also a contributor to the increased prevalence of global related diseases (Sterling et al. 2020). In fact, alcohol abuse has been cited to be one of the underlying causes for the increase in alcohol related medical conditions and a contributory factor to many more illnesses. Social isolation and related stress issues caused by the COVID-19 pandemic have contributed to the increases in alcohol consumption. Individuals with underlying related comorbidities are at greater risk of death and serious illness than healthy sections of the population who abuse alcohol. Further to this, alcohol misuse is related to both unintentional and intentional injuries (NIAAA 2021). Information about the disease risks of alcohol abuse has helped inform policy makers in the promotion of sensible alcohol consumption guidelines. However, the guidelines during the recent pandemic have been compromised in relation to the recoded increases in alcohol consumption over the COVID-19 period (Steffen et al. 2021). Further to this, and in addition to the increased disease risks that can potentially harm alcohol abusers, severe alcohol consumption can also have an impact on the health status of drinkers while causing social harm to the drinker's family and friends (Moss 2013). The results of studies indicating social harm and medical damage to individuals during the pandemic need to be considered urgently. The findings highlight the need for the urgent development of effective prevention strategies to reduce the burden, suffering, and costs, linked with greater alcohol consumption particularly pre and post the COVID-19 pandemic. Individuals with related comorbidities need to be extra vigilant in relation to their alcohol use. Alcohol accelerates the disease process, and in compromised individuals and patient populations, alcohol abuse will be a contributory factor to their premature demise and or serious illness.

Not only health but economies suffer as much from alcohol abuse as its detrimental effects on health, affecting not only families, but communities, institutions, and individuals of all ages. Young people who drink too much are impeding their development, while impacting on the country's ability to face economic challenges in the future. In families with alcohol-dependent members, health care costs are twice as high as in families without alcohol abusers, and up to half of all emergency room visits are due to alcoholism (Burke 1988). In response to COVID19, drinking practices have changed considerably. People drink at home instead of in bars and restaurants. While bar and restaurant sales have fallen, off-premises sales, such as ecommerce and retail stores, have grown significantly. US online sales, for instance, increased by 234%. There is a heavy toll on society, the economy, and individuals resulting from harmful alcohol consumption. According to the projection for the next 30 years, illnesses and injuries caused by consuming more than 1.5 drinks per day for men and 1 drink per day for women will cause life expectancy to be 0.9 years shorter in OECD countries. Health expenditures will be responsible for approximately 2.4% of GDP, while participation and productivity among the workforce will be reduced by 1.6% (OECD 2021). OECD countries report that drinking more than 1/1.5 drinks per day increases the likelihood of a number of diseases and adds USD 61 per capita to annual health care costs, adjusted for purchasing power parity. Over the course of the analysis, the total cost of treating these diseases is USD purchasing power parity 138 billion per year across all the OECD countries included in recent analysis. The current health expenditure in Australia is equivalent to this amount, while the current health expenditure in Belgium is more than double that amount (OECD 2021).

In summary, we hope that the content of this paper will stimulate debate and raise awareness of the increased alcohol abuse problems during and post the COVID-19 pandemic. The content provided here outlines the detrimental effects of alcohol abuse and suggests reasons for increases in consumption during the pandemic. The paper also comments on the risk factors and economic costs associated with alcohol abuse in healthy individuals and individuals with underlying comorbidities. In addition, the paper also discusses the effects of excessive alcohol consumption on psychological parameters and implications for social harm and societal disengagement. We hope that the contents of this paper will provide information that will invigorate local governmental and global health organizations to produce intervention strategies, and innovative new policies and policy amendments (especially online selling, ecommerce, and retail stores) to alleviate this risk and associated economic burdens.

Author Contributions: J.S.B. wrote the paper, J.S.B. and R.S. designed the study. D.T. and Y.G. contributed to discussion and editing. All authors have read and agreed to the published version of the manuscript.

Funding: This research received no external funding.

Institutional Review Board Statement: Not applicable.

Informed Consent Statement: Not applicable.

Data Availability Statement: Not applicable.

Acknowledgments: This paper was prepared from the presentation on idea presented in the symposium "Transnational and Transdisciplinary Lessons of COVID-19 From the Perspective of Risk and Management".

Conflicts of Interest: The authors declare no conflict of interest.

References

Burke, Terrence R. 1988. The Economic Impact of Alcohol Abuse and Alcoholism. *Public Health Reports* 103: 564–68. [PubMed]

Clay, James M., and Matthew O. Parker. 2020. Alcohol use and misuse during the COVID-19 pandemic: A potential public health crisis? *The Lancet Public Health* 5: e259. [CrossRef]

Gama, Ana, Ana Rita Pedroa, Maria João Leote de Carvalho, Ana Esteves Guerreiro, Vera Duarte, Jorge Quintas, Andreia Matias, Ines Keygnaert, and Sónia Dias. 2020. Domestic Violence during the COVID-19 Pandemic in Portugal. *Portuguese Journal of Public Health* 38: 32–40. [CrossRef]

Grossman, Elyse R., Sara E. Benjamin-Neelon, and Susan Sonnenschein. 2020. Alcohol Consumption during the COVID-19 Pandemic: A Cross-Sectional Survey of US Adults. *International Journal of Environmental Research and Public Health* 17: 9189. [CrossRef] [PubMed]

Hou, Wai Kai, Tatia Mei-chun Lee, Li Liang, Tsz W. Li, Huinan Liu, Horace Tong, Menachem Ben-Ezra, and Robin Goodwin. 2021. Psychiatric symptoms and behavioral adjustment during the COVID-19 pandemic: Evidence from two population-representative cohorts. *Translational Psychiatry* 11: 174. [CrossRef] [PubMed]

Kuitunen-Paul, Sören, and Michael Roerecke. 2018. Alcohol Use Disorders Identification Test (AUDIT) and mortality risk: A systematic review and meta-analysis. *Journal of Epidemiology and Community Health* 72: 856–63. [CrossRef] [PubMed]

Moss, Howard B. 2013. The Impact of Alcohol on Society: A Brief Overview. *Social Work in Public Health* 28: 175–77. [CrossRef] [PubMed]

NIAAA National Institute on Alcohol Abuse and Alcoholism. 2021. Available online: https://www.niaaa.nih.gov/publications/brochures-and-fact-sheets/alcohol-facts-and-statistics (accessed on 25 September 2021).

OECD. 2021. *Preventing Harmful Alcohol Use*. OECD Health Policy Studies. Paris: OECD, ISBN 9789264594043.

Pollard, Michael S., Joan S. Tucker, and Harold D. Green Jr. 2020. Changes in Adult Alcohol Use and Consequences During the COVID-19 Pandemic in the US. *JAMA Network Open* 3: e2022942. [CrossRef] [PubMed]

Rehm, Jürgen, Carolin Kilian, Carina Ferreira-Borges, David Jernigan, Maristela Monteiro, Charles D. H. Parry, Zila M. Sanchez, and Jakob Manthey. 2020. Alcohol use in times of the COVID-19: Implications for monitoring and policy. *Drug and Alcohol Review* 39: 301–4. [CrossRef] [PubMed]

Steffen, Julius, Jenny Schlichtiger, Bruno C. Huber, and Stefan Brunner. 2021. Altered alcohol consumption during COVID-19 pandemic lockdown. *Journal of Nutrition* 20: 44. [CrossRef] [PubMed]

Sterling, Stacy A., Vanessa A. Palzes, Yun Lu, Andrea H. Kline-Simon, Sujaya Parthasarathy, Thekla Ross, Joseph Elson, Constance Weisner, Clara Maxim, and Felicia W. Chi. 2020. Associations Between Medical Conditions and Alcohol Consumption Levels in an Adult Primary Care Population. *JAMA Network Open* 3: e204687. [CrossRef] [PubMed]

World Health Organisation Alcohol. 2018. Available online: https://www.who.int/news-room/fact-sheets/detail/alcohol (accessed on 25 September 2021).

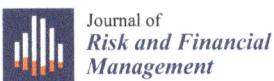

Editorial

COVID-19 Impact on the Sport Sector Economy and Athletic Performance

Huw D. Wiltshire [1,*], Rashmi Supriya [2] and Julien S. Baker [2]

1. School of Sport and Health Sciences, Cardiff Metropolitan University, Cardiff CF5 2YB, UK
2. Centre for Health and Exercise Science Research, Hong Kong Baptist University, Hong Kong 999077, China; rashmisupriya@hkbu.edu.hk (R.S.); jsbaker@hkbu.edu.hk (J.S.B.)
* Correspondence: hwiltshire@cardiffmet.ac.uk

Citation: Wiltshire, Huw D., Rashmi Supriya, and Julien S. Baker. 2022. COVID-19 Impact on the Sport Sector Economy and Athletic Performance. *Journal of Risk and Financial Management* 15: 173. https://doi.org/10.3390/jrfm15040173

Received: 12 March 2022
Accepted: 1 April 2022
Published: 9 April 2022

Publisher's Note: MDPI stays neutral with regard to jurisdictional claims in published maps and institutional affiliations.

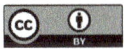

Copyright: © 2022 by the authors. Licensee MDPI, Basel, Switzerland. This article is an open access article distributed under the terms and conditions of the Creative Commons Attribution (CC BY) license (https://creativecommons.org/licenses/by/4.0/).

As COVID-19 continues to impact global health, and educational, financial, commercial institutions, sport, in particular, has not been spared. A number of major games, fixtures and competitions have been cancelled or postponed, disrupting governing bodies, organisers, teams, and athletic performers and preventing the continuous streaming of live sport, something the global sporting audience has become accustomed to (Deloitte 2020). A detailed article entitled '2020: The Year in Sports When Everyone Lost' appeared in the New York Times on 13 December. The article reported losses of USD 13 billion in the US sporting leagues, while some of Europe's largest football clubs reported revenue losses exceeding EUR 1 billion. The outcomes were equally disastrous in other sub-sectors of sport, including Wimbledon and the Olympics (Sato et al. 2020; Skinner and Smith 2021).

In March 2020, the World Health Organisation (WHO) defined the coronavirus disease 2019 (COVID-19) as a pandemic. The current global context indicates a volume of 246,357,468 confirmed COVID-19 cases with a concomitant fatality trend of 4,995,412 (WHO 2021). Regarding cost, it is estimated that the United Kingdom would experience a drop in revenue of GBP 8.6 billion, which would equate to approximately 17% of the total decline across Europe. In broader terms, the impact of COVID-19 across the sporting sector in Europe would be likely to reflect a reduction of around GBP 52 billion in GDP and a loss of over a million employees. This has been highlighted by the economic pressure exerted by the pandemic on elite basketball: "while the cost of the season resumption was reportedly $150 million—and the league had lost more than $1 billion in revenue due to the pandemic—restarting the season also saved the league 'hundreds of millions' in TV revenue and saved players $600 million in salary" (Hindman et al. 2021). The closure of local venues and facilities in conjunction with fierce social distancing have led to the cessation of social and participatory sport in cities (Mastromartino et al. 2020). Professional sport and its competitive leagues also suffered via low cash influx without revenue from fans, such as gate receipts, concessions, merchandise, and sponsorships, although the worst losses came from decreased broadcasting. Although the NFL (National Football League) and its franchises managed to overcome the financial chasm left by the pandemic's estimated but ongoing USD 6 billion impact, few other sporting organizations had either the reserves or state support to compensate for the losses. Sponsors have been damaged, especially those who rely on exposure from events, endorsements from players, and retail sales (Dašić et al. 2020). Adidas, for example, has closed all of its retail locations worldwide, and their sponsorship deals have crumbled in the void created by closing events and competitions (Skinner and Smith 2021). Following the COVID-19 pandemic lockdowns in 2020, many companies will not be able to survive without public support. Sport companies face a significant threat of survival from a single-year recession of 23%. This will impact massively on some of the policy proposals applied to the field of sport economics. For instance: (a) *Relief packages to boost the sport sector:* For the sport sector to be boosted during pandemics, short-term relief packages will be needed. In the UK, this was accomplished through the National Lottery. For example, the government and the National Lottery provided funding of GBP 195 million to the sport and physical activity sector in response to the pandemic, which ranged from providing financial support to local sports clubs to finding new and innovative ways to keep people active and reopen businesses after the pandemic (Kokolakakis et al. 2021); (b)*Tax Breaks:* Tax breaks for events that are major tourist attractions can indirectly boost tax revenues since sports are related to broader economic activities such as tourism and accommodation. Tax breaks can be a way to reinvigorate the sport industry (Sport England 2020); and (c) *Reinvesting Sport Related Budgetary Surpluses:* Numerous economic studies have shown that grassroots sport and consumer demand for sport contribute positively to public finances (Department for Digital Culture and Account 2018). Sport facilities that are inclusive and family-friendly can attract latent participants and be a motivating factor for non-participants. Supporting sports participation could be improved by government policy by reinvesting net broadcasting revenues in grassroots sports and by distributing funding from elite leagues to lower tiers. A higher number of participants, especially new ones who are more likely to purchase sports consumables, leads to a higher demand for sporting goods and services, leading to greater budgetary surpluses (Kokolakakis and Lera-Lopez 2020).

There also exists a fundamental need to examine the effects of prolonged quarantine on athletes' health and performance (Grazioli et al. 2020). It is evident that during a confinement period, it may be incredibly challenging for athletes to undertake routine training that would typically occur with teammates within a performance environment led by a range of coaches and scientific experts (Tayech et al. 2020). In professional basketball, researchersadministered a six-question confidential survey to more than two hundred NBA players. Their research suggested: COVID-19 affected the NBA players' ability to maintain peak performance levels; NBA players displayed consistent levels of calmness during the pandemic, indicating excellent coping mechanisms; there was no indication of mental wellbeing being negatively affected by the pandemic; NBA players were in receipt of a variety of meaningful resources and support from their NBA franchises; NBA players' most prominent concern related to the uncertainty of returning to play; and, across a range of franchises, NBA players were maintaining fitness, connecting with friends and family, and researching business opportunities during time off. An argument was presented that COVID-19 is more detrimental than a traditional off season on physical performance (Grazioli et al. 2020). This research work on Brazilian professional soccer players found that body composition, counter movement jump (CMJ) and sprint performance were significantly impaired after sixty-three days of quarantine compared with a regular off-season period of twenty-four days. Substantial reductions were also found in certain physical capabilities, such as hamstring eccentric strength (i.e., ranging from 1 to 11% and from 2 to 27% of decreases in absolute and relative strength, respectively) and cardiorespiratory fitness (i.e., assessed through the YO-YO test for soccer, ranging from 1 to 21% of decreases in intermittent total distance). After five months of lockdown in the National Football League in 2011, Achilles tendon ruptures increased by 500% compared with the same period in regular seasons (Myer et al. 2011). Three key reasons have been identified as to why lockdown may be more detrimental: it does not reflect a traditional off-season due to the physiological and psychological restrictions of confinement; the following pre-season will be affected by congested preparation and, potentially, more susceptibility to injury; and, in a condensed preparation phase, the acute–chronic workload demands will directly increase risk injury (Bisciotti et al. 2020).

From a physiological perspective, quarantine and confinement can reflect an adverse element of detraining without the necessary support mechanisms for athletes. The physiological effects of detraining from the cardiovascular, cardiorespiratory, musculo-skeletal and miscellaneous perspectives have also been outlined (Mulcahey et al. 2021). A consistent practical implication for detraining is connected to negative changes in body composition and body mass. With an accompanying potential for impaired functional capacity of the neuromuscular and cardiovascular systems, this can in turn create a regression in strength, speed, flexibility and endurance outputs (Bosquet et al. 2013). Research analysing the psychological impact of the pandemic has exposed a clear detrimental impact upon psychological health associated with social distancing (Taylor 2019). Disruption due to COVID-19 carries a clear psychological impact due to athletes having no previous experience of pandemic-caused confinement. Ultimately, "COVID-19 has significant physical and mental effects on athletes including physical deconditioning, altered sleep patterns, worsening nutrition, uncertainty on RTS and feelings of depression" (Pillay et al. 2020). A key focal point for elite coaches and athletes is the analysis of confined training methodologies. It has been argued that basic levels of physical activity during confinement could improve the athletes' quality of life (Slimani et al. 2020). Research highlighted that training during home confinement tended to concentrate on strength, power, and muscular endurance exercises, general physical preparation (e.g., aerobic training on a range of ergometers), and stretching, amongst other isolation-limited activities (Tayech et al. 2020). As such, "countries, communities, and individuals must be prepared to cope in the longer-term with both the demands and the consequences of living with such essential containment and prevention measures" (Skegg et al. 2021). The broad aim of introducing COVID-19 preventative measures to athletes is to lower risk symptoms, prevent transmission, and limit the total numbers affected. Designed carefully, this will allow for the safe return to athletic participation whilst also minimising the number of COVID-19-related interruptions to training. This objective can assist in reducing any adverse physiological effects that may impair an athlete's ability to return to pre-COVID-19 levels in the short and long term (Mulcahey et al. 2021). It is imperative that specific training and injury prevention programmes be developed, with careful load monitoring, in order to limit the decrement in physiological changes, both central and peripheral, of the aerobic system (Bisciotti et al. 2020). It has been suggested that athletes initiate a conservative approach, limiting training sessions to less than sixty minutes and at an intensity of less than 80% of the maximum ability during this time to prevent COVID-19 (Toresdahl and Asif 2020). Key research data indicate that enhancing balance training improves speed, strength and power (Makhlouf et al. 2018). Broadly speaking, athletes can use confinement to focus on the weaker aspects of their physical and psychological performance, completing relevant recovery activities to allow for super compensation. Global digital usage trends highlight the fact that there are 4.66 billion active internet users worldwide, which equates to 59.5 percent of the global population. Moreover, 92.6 percent (4.32 billion) access the internet via mobile devices. Further patterns in usage have increased during COVID-19 (Clements 2020). Elite athletes will need to embrace online digital platforms to enhance decision making and problem-based learning. In addition, social media can be used to disseminate knowledge and provide athlete and coach feedback whilst sharing positive messaging and behaviours. Finally, media education can be explored to frame the opportunities linked to COVID-19 confinement athletic training (Tayech et al. 2020). Appropriate sports nutrition improves performance, reduces fatigue, and limits the risk of illness and injury; it also allows athletes to optimise their training and recover more quickly (Thomas et al. 2016). A balanced, healthy diet is critical for the maintenance of immune function, especially important during COVID-19 confinement. It is critical that athletes consume foods rich in vitamins A, C, E, B6, and B12, zinc, and iron (Naja and Hamadeh 2020).

In conclusion, the pandemic has created financial burdens for sport providers and the media. COVID-19 has also impacted individual athletes' potential to generate revenue and provide for their families. The risk of transmission has had a massive impact on sports performance for competitors and spectators. This has resulted in increased anxiety and social confinement. Further to this, the closure of venues and facilities has contributed to the decline in health of the general population. These scenarios need reversing urgently post pandemic to provide entertainment for spectators, revenue generation for sports organisations and the media, and increased health status for the general population.

Author Contributions: Conceptualization, H.D.W. and J.S.B.; writing—original draft preparation, H.D.W., R.S. and J.S.B.; writing—review and editing, R.S. and J.S.B. All authors have read and agreed to the published version of the manuscript.

Funding: This research received no external funding.

Acknowledgments: This paper was prepared from the presentation on idea presented in the symposium "Transnational and Transdisciplinary Lessons of COVID-19 From the Perspective of Risk and Management".

Conflicts of Interest: The authors declare no conflict of interest.

References

Bisciotti, Gian Nicola, Cristiano Eirale, Alessandro Corsini, Christophe Baudot, Gerard Saillant, and Hakim Chalabi. 2020. Return to Football Training and Competition after Lockdown Caused by the COVID-19 Pandemic: Medical Recommendations. *Biology of Sport* 37: 313–19. [CrossRef] [PubMed]

Bosquet, Laurent, Nicolas Berryman, Olivier Dupuy, S. Mekary, D. Arvisais, Louis Bherer, and I. Mujika. 2013. Effect of Training Cessation on Muscular Performance: A Meta-Analysis. *Scandinavian Journal of Medicine & Science in Sports* 23: e140–49. [CrossRef]

Clements, John M. 2020. Knowledge and Behaviors Toward COVID-19 Among US Residents During the Early Days of the Pandemic: Cross-Sectional Online Questionnaire. *JMIR Public Health and Surveillance* 6: e19161. [CrossRef] [PubMed]

Dašić, Dejan, Miloš Tošić, and Velimir Deletić. 2020. The Impact of the COVID-19 Pandemic on the Advertising and Sponsorship Industry in Sport. *Bizinfo Blace* 11: 105–16. [CrossRef]

Deloitte. 2020. *Understanding the Impact of COVID-19 on the Sports Industry*. London: Deloitte.

Department for Digital Culture and Account. 2018. *2016 Department for Digital Culture, M.& S. UK Sport Satellite Account, 2016 Provisional*. London: Department for Digital Culture and Account.

Grazioli, Rafael, Irineu Loturco, Bruno M. Baroni, Gabriel S. Oliveira, Vasyl Saciura, Everton Vanoni, Rafael Dias, Filipe Veeck, Ronei S. Pinto, and Eduardo L. Cadore. 2020. Coronavirus Disease-19 Quarantine Is More Detrimental Than Traditional Off-Season on Physical Conditioning of Professional Soccer Players. *Journal of Strength and Conditioning Research* 34: 3316–20. [CrossRef] [PubMed]

Hindman, Lauren C., Nefertiti A. Walker, and Kwame J. A. Agyemang. 2021. Bounded Rationality or Bounded Morality? The National Basketball Association Response to COVID-19. *European Sport Management Quarterly* 21: 333–49. [CrossRef]

Kokolakakis, Themistocles, and Fernando Lera-Lopez. 2020. Sport Promotion through Sport Mega-Events. An Analysis for Types of Olympic Sports in London 2012. *International Journal of Environmental Research and Public Health* 17: 6193. [CrossRef] [PubMed]

Kokolakakis, Themis, Fernando Lera-Lopez, and Girish Ramchandani. 2021. Measuring the Economic Impact of COVID-19 on the UK's Leisure and Sport during the 2020 Lockdown. *Sustainability* 13: 13865. [CrossRef]

Makhlouf, Issam, Anis Chaouachi, Mehdi Chaouachi, Aymen Ben Othman, Urs Granacher, and David G. Behm. 2018. Combination of Agility and Plyometric Training Provides Similar Training Benefits as Combined Balance and Plyometric Training in Young Soccer Players. *Frontiers in Physiology* 9: 1611. [CrossRef]

Mastromartino, Brandon, Walker J. Ross, Henry Wear, and Michael L. Naraine. 2020. Thinking Outside the 'Box': A Discussion of Sports Fans, Teams, and the Environment in the Context of COVID-19. *Sport in Society* 23: 1707–23. [CrossRef]

Mulcahey, Mary K., Arianna L. Gianakos, Angela Mercurio, Scott Rodeo, and Karen M. Sutton. 2021. Sports Medicine Considerations During the COVID-19 Pandemic. *The American Journal of Sports Medicine* 49: 512–21. [CrossRef] [PubMed]

Myer, Gregory D., Avery D. Faigenbaum, Chad E. Cherny, Robert S. Heidt, and Timothy E. Hewett. 2011. Did the NFL Lockout Expose the Achilles Heel of Competitive Sports? *Journal of Orthopaedic & Sports Physical Therapy* 41: 702–5. [CrossRef]

Naja, Farah, and Rena Hamadeh. 2020. Nutrition amid the COVID-19 Pandemic: A Multi-Level Framework for Action. *European Journal of Clinical Nutrition* 74: 1117–21. [CrossRef] [PubMed]

Pillay, Lervasen, Dina C. Christa Janse van Rensburg, Audrey Jansen van Rensburg, Dimakatso A. Ramagole, Louis Holtzhausen, H. Paul Dijkstra, and Tanita Cronje. 2020. Nowhere to Hide: The Significant Impact of Coronavirus Disease 2019 (COVID-19) Measures on Elite and Semi-Elite South African Athletes. *Journal of Science and Medicine in Sport* 23: 670–79. [CrossRef]

Sato, Shintaro, Daichi Oshimi, Yoshifumi Bizen, and Rei Saito. 2020. The COVID-19 Outbreak and Public Perceptions of Sport Events in Japan. *Managing Sport and Leisure* 27: 1–6. [CrossRef]

Skegg, David, Peter Gluckman, Geoffrey Boulton, Heide Hackmann, Salim S. Abdool Karim, Peter Piot, and Christiane Woopen. 2021. Future Scenarios for the COVID-19 Pandemic. *The Lancet* 397: 777–78. [CrossRef]

Skinner, James, and Aaron C. T. Smith. 2021. Introduction: Sport and COVID-19: Impacts and Challenges for the Future (Volume 1). *European Sport Management Quarterly* 21: 323–32. [CrossRef]

Slimani, Maamer, Armin Paravlic, Faten Mbarek, Nicola L. Bragazzi, and David Tod. 2020. The Relationship Between Physical Activity and Quality of Life During the Confinement Induced by COVID-19 Outbreak: A Pilot Study in Tunisia. *Frontiers in Psychology* 11: 1–5. [CrossRef]

Sport England. 2020. *Other Ways to Generate Funding*. London: Sport England.

Tayech, Amel, Mohamed Arbi Mejri, Issam Makhlouf, Ameni Mathlouthi, David G. Behm, and Anis Chaouachi. 2020. Second Wave of COVID-19 Global Pandemic and Athletes' Confinement: Recommendations to Better Manage and Optimize the Modified Lifestyle. *International Journal of Environmental Research and Public Health* 17: 8385. [CrossRef]

Taylor, Steven. 2019. *The Psychology of Pandemics: Preparing for the Next Global Outbreak of Infectious Disease. The Psychology of Pandemics: Preparing for the next Global Outbreak of Infectious Disease*. Newcastle upon Tyne: Cambridge Scholars Publishing, ISBN 1-5275-3959-8 (Hardcover); 978-1-5275-3959-4 (Hardcover).

Thomas, D. Travis, Kelly Anne Erdman, and Louise M. Burke. 2016. Position of the Academy of Nutrition and Dietetics, Dietitians of Canada, and the American College of Sports Medicine: Nutrition and Athletic Performance. *Journal of the Academy of Nutrition and Dietetics* 116: 501–28. [CrossRef]

Toresdahl, Brett G., and Irfan M. Asif. 2020. Coronavirus Disease 2019 (COVID-19): Considerations for the Competitive Athlete. *Sports Health: A Multidisciplinary Approach* 12: 221–24. [CrossRef] [PubMed]

WHO. 2021. *WHO Coronavirus Disease (COVID-19) Dashboard*. Geneva: WHO.

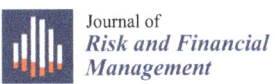

Editorial

COVID-19: Barriers to Physical Activity in Older Adults, a Decline in Health or Economy?

Jiao Jiao [1], Rashmi Supriya [2], Bik C. Chow [1,2,*], Julien S. Baker [2,3,*], Frédéric Dutheil [4], Yang Gao [2,3], Sze-Hoi Chan [1], Wei Liang [3], Feifei Li [3] and Dan Tao [2]

[1] Dr. Stephen Hui Research Centre for Physical Recreation and Wellness, Faculty of Social Sciences, Hong Kong Baptist University, Hong Kong, China; jojojiao@hkbu.edu.hk (J.J.); anthonychan714@gmail.com (S.-H.C.)

[2] Department of Sport, Physical Education and Health, Faculty of Social Sciences, Hong Kong Baptist University, Hong Kong, China; rashmisupriya@hkbu.edu.hk (R.S.); gaoyang@hkbu.edu.hk (Y.G.); emma0514@hkbu.edu.hk (D.T.)

[3] Centre for Health and Exercise Science Research, Department of Sport, Physical Education and Health, Hong Kong Baptist University, Hong Kong, China; wliang1020@hkbu.edu.hk (W.L.); lifeifei@hkbu.edu.hk (F.L.)

[4] Université Clermont Auvergne, CNRS, LaPSCo, Physiological and Psychosocial Stress, University Hospital of Clermont-Ferrand, CHU Clermont-Ferrand, Occupational and Environmental Medicine, 63000 Clermont-Ferrand, France; fred_dutheil@yahoo.fr

* Correspondence: bchow@hkbu.edu.hk (B.C.C.); jsbaker@hkbu.edu.hk (J.S.B.)

Citation: Jiao, Jiao, Rashmi Supriya, Bik C. Chow, Julien S. Baker, Frédéric Dutheil, Yang Gao, Sze-Hoi Chan, Wei Liang, Feifei Li, and Dan Tao. 2022. COVID-19: Barriers to Physical Activity in Older Adults, a Decline in Health or Economy? *Journal of Risk and Financial Management* 15: 51. https://doi.org/10.3390/jrfm15020051

Received: 8 December 2021
Accepted: 21 January 2022
Published: 23 January 2022

Publisher's Note: MDPI stays neutral with regard to jurisdictional claims in published maps and institutional affiliations.

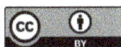

Copyright: © 2022 by the authors. Licensee MDPI, Basel, Switzerland. This article is an open access article distributed under the terms and conditions of the Creative Commons Attribution (CC BY) license (https://creativecommons.org/licenses/by/4.0/).

Since spring 2020, in response to the global threat of the Coronavirus Disease 2019 (COVID-19) pandemic, several governments implemented emergency policies and regulations to prevent further transmission of the disease (Portegijs et al. 2021). Social distancing, isolation or lock-downs have been adopted to control the transmission and protect citizens. These regulations involve typically restricting the mobility of citizens and the closure of activity destinations. Although the measures could "flatten the curve" of new cases and minimize the infection rates, the restrictions have also had significant impacts on citizens' health and well-being due to the amplification of the barriers to physical activity (PA). The impacts may be more obvious and impactful to vulnerable populations, namely, the elderly and those with chronic medical conditions and individuals with sedentary behaviors (Marashi et al. 2021). Evidence has shown that the decline in PA could represent an increased risk of developing functional limitations and daily living disabilities (Tak et al. 2013), chronic diseases such as cardiovascular disease (Hupin et al. 2015), obesity (Zbrońska and Mędrela-Kuder 2018), cognitive decline (Shah et al. 2017), dementia (Guure et al. 2017), depression (Schuch et al. 2018) and the rate of all-cause mortality (Hupin et al. 2015). In contrast, there are numerous benefits for improving PA, which have been thoroughly reported in previous studies. The level of and engagement in PA are also associated with the economy of a country, especially from the aspects of healthcare and medication. According to a previous report from Australia, almost 7% of Australia's health burden was attributed to physical inactivity, with the main contributors being ischemic heart disease (51%), type 2 diabetes (20%) and stroke (14%) (Begg et al. 2007). The diseases usually occur in elderly adults. This indicates that elderly populations would be badly affected by COVID-19 but would also gain the most benefit from increased levels of PA. The increased PA levels would result in a decreased occurrence of the disease and facilitate a decline in future economic demands of healthcare and medication.

According to previous studies prior to COVID-19, there were some existing physical barriers for PA participation for the elderly including physical limitations such as discomfort and different kinds of pain. In addition, psychosocial barriers such as lack of motivation and lack of enjoyment also exist, in conjunction with other numerous barriers such as environmental factors and social support, etc. (Portegijs et al. 2020). During the COVID-19 epidemic, the existing barriers have been widely amplified. Many governments have implemented measures such as lockdowns to control the spread of Severe Acute Respiratory Syndrome Coronavirus 2 (SARS-CoV-2). These measures have resulted in public sports and recreational facilities being forced to close. Now, as communities are returning to normal activities and more people are in the public domain more often, physical distancing is used as a common approach globally to ensure physical space between people in public areas. The rationale behind social distancing is to minimize the virus spread by avoiding crowds, group gatherings, and refraining from individual contact with one another (Nilsen et al. 2020). However, these policies have brought about an increase in sedentary behavior and relational distancing, which has resulted in a general norm for the increased physical inactivity of citizens. The impact is more apparent among vulnerable groups, such as the elderly and those with chronic medical conditions. The situation of city-wide lockdowns or restrictive access to public sports facilities has forced individuals to change hobbies and habits, and the elderly have been reported to associate with decreased activity during the COVID-19 pandemic (Suzuki et al. 2020). In addition, Yuta Suzuki's research team (Suzuki et al. 2020) found that elderly people in a relevantly more dormant state faced another physical obstacle that related to the changes in daily transportation needs.

Considering its impact on health, the environmental limitations restricted PA levels, leading to the deterioration of function or cognitive decline, which would adversely affect PA levels. As reported by Yamada's research team (Yamada et al. 2020), the total PA time decreased by 65 min per week across frailty and robust groups of older adults in Japan during the first 3 months of the COVID-19 pandemic. The decreasing rates recorded were 30% and 36.4% in frail and robust older adults, respectively. The PA decrease may indicate a deteriorating trend of physical function and disability in the future (Yamada et al. 2020). Not only physically, the COVID-19 pandemic has also induced dramatic changes in psychosocial status. The elderly and people with severe comorbidities are particularly vulnerable to the adverse consequences of COVID-19. This issue may cause considerable fear among the elderly and exaggerate other related psychological problems including increases in anxiety, irritability and excessive stress (Dubey et al. 2020). These psychological impacts on the elderly may automatically transform into a sense of self-protection awareness by confining themselves to home because they have increased concerns about being infected when contacting others. The contact may occur with close relations and friends during gatherings indoors or with strangers in crowded places in public areas. Hence, psychological stresses such as fear and anxiety are potentially perceived barriers to outdoor activities. The COVID-19 pandemic has provided a situation where a paradoxical loop has developed. This paradox relates to the fact that elderly populations are unable to conduct physical activities due to the psychological stresses or closure of faculties, simultaneously; they are unable to relieve their psychological stresses through physical activities. A summary of the barriers to physical activity of older adults amplified by the COVID-19 pandemic and the relevant effects to elderly's health and economy has been summarized in Figure 1.

In relation to the economy, healthcare and hospitalization costs may increase with increases in the age of populations and their aggravation of diseases. When the elderly become less active, they have more risk of sarcopenia, depression, dementia and Alzheimer's disease and are a majority group who are subjected to multi-morbidity with implications for proper medical care and social service support. According to a study published in 2016 examining data from the United States in 2014, non-institutionalized adults aged 50 years old and greater cost a staggering USD 860 billion annually in healthcare. This figure is amazing when we consider that four out of five of the most costly chronic conditions among the elderly can be prevented or managed by PA (Watson et al. 2016). Similarly, research conducted in the pre-pandemic period in Australia illustrated that, if the prevalence of physical inactivity in adults experienced a reduction of 10%, this would result in 6000 fewer incident cases of the disease, 2000 fewer deaths and 25,000 fewer disability-adjusted life years, which may confer a reduction of AUD 96 million in health sector costs (Cadilhac et al. 2011). Two recent studies during the COVID-19 pandemic have illustrated similar concepts that billions of dollars in global health-related expenditure could be saved by improving the level of PA (Hafner et al. 2019; Hafner et al. 2020), since regular PA is associated with lower onset rates of different chronic diseases, such as obesity, hypertension, diabetes and dementia, etc. (Baker et al. 2021; Guure et al. 2017), when people progress in age. Although it is unrealistic to expect immediately converting health costs to savings when people become sufficiently active (Stephenson et al. 2000), the cost of pharmaceuticals might be reduced in the short term. For example, blood pressure could be reduced by 3–5 mmHg if individuals began to conduct regular moderate PA; using this scenario, the cost for antihypertensive medication would be reduced. From a long-term perspective, a large amount of savings from the reduction in cost of health care, hospitalization and medication because of physical inactivity could be used for individual services followed by economically supporting the government and healthcare providers, which would further benefit the entire society. Taking an example of Hong Kong, whose population is ageing, the total health spending from 1989/90 to 2019/20 grew at an average annual rate of 5.6% in real terms, faster than the corresponding 3.4% increase in the gross domestic product (GDP) during the same period. As a result, total health expenditure as a percentage of the GDP increased from 3.6% in 1989/90 to 6.8% in 2019/20 (Food and Health Bureau 2021) and is expected to continuously increase in the coming years. Even after the resumption of the world economy when the COVID-19 pandemic ends, the economic impacts of physical inactivity due to the barriers amplified by COVID-19 would remain. If this sedentary lifestyle in the elderly continues, the number of health-related expenditures could increase even more, which would consequently result in a heavier burden to the government in the future, as 53% of the current health expenditure was paid via government schemes, and only 30% was by household out-of-pocket payment in 2019/20 (Food and Health Bureau 2021).

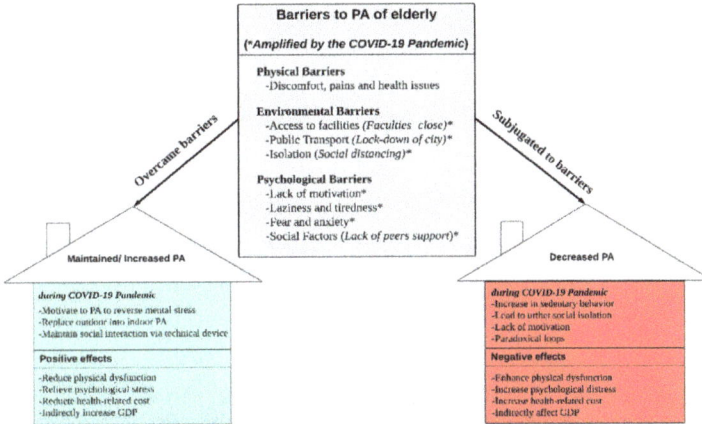

Figure 1. Summary of the barriers to physical activity of older adults amplified by the COVID-19 pandemic and the relevant effects to elderly's health and economy.

Therefore, in order to maintain health and safeguard the economy, a further initiative to overcome barriers to physical activity includes tools such as online exercise videos, apps, online platforms and telehealth media. These tools are not limited by environmental barriers and are fundamental international recommendations for maintaining mental health and physical health during the COVID-19 quarantine. There are various online group exercise classes that could be freely provided to the elderly. As recommended by The WHO Regional Office for Europe, following "online exercise classes" would be a positive way to be active as this method has demonstrated positive relevance to PA during self-isolation (Stay Physically Active during Self-Quarantine 2020). In addition, these methods for PA can help the elderly avoid the risk of being infected and encourage them to continue their physical activities within their own comfort zones and the safety of their homes. In this

COVID-19 era, older people should be made aware of web-based applications that can keep them physically and mentally fit. Web-based applications that are available for older adults include Bold, Silver Sneakers Go, Britain's National Health Service, Calm, C25K and Healthline (The Best Health and Fitness Apps for Seniors). Furthermore, we think future healthcare provision will be reliant on artificial intelligence (AI). In fact, the era of AI medication seems inevitable. Patients can use AI chatbots at home to keep track of their health plans at the simplest level. It may be possible to remove anxiety and confusion associated with seniors by using artificial intelligence applications that remind them when to take their medication, when to see their doctors and even when to eat. Social robots powered by AI can go beyond this by providing senior citizens with some level of companionship. Social robots can also nudge self-care behaviors by tailoring their engagement (Greulich-Smith 2020). In summary, despite putting the blame on governments, it is our responsibility as citizens to make use of the available technologies to protect not just the health of our elderly but also our economy. These technologies need to be realized soon and made freely available. This development would facilitate increases in PA while reducing the economic and medical burdens associated with physical inactivity.

Author Contributions: Conceptualization, J.J., B.C.C. and S.-H.C.; writing—original draft preparation, J.J. and S.-H.C.; writing—review and editing, B.C.C., J.S.B. and F.D.; literature search and review, Y.G., W.L., D.T., R.S. and F.L. All authors have read and agreed to the published version of the manuscript.

Funding: This research received no external funding.

Acknowledgments: We acknowledge Gordon Cheung for his technical and administrative support to this paper.

Conflicts of Interest: The authors declare no conflict of interest.

References

Baker, Julien S., Alistair Cole, Dan Tao, Feifei Li, Wei Liang, Jojo Jiao, Yang Gao, and Rashmi Supriya. 2021. The preventive role of exercise on the physiological, psychological, and psychophysiological parameters of coronavirus 2 (SARS-CoV-2): A mini review. *Journal of Risk and Financial Management* 14: 476. [CrossRef]

Begg, Stephen, Vos Theo, Barker Bridget, Stevenson Chris, Stanley Lucy, and Lopenz Alan. 2007. The Burden of Disease and Injury in Australia 2003. Available online: https://www.aihw.gov.au/reports/burden-of-disease/burden-of-disease-injury-australia-2003 (accessed on 20 October 2021).

Cadilhac, Dominique A., Toby B. Cumming, Lauren Sheppard, Dora C. Pearce, Rob Carter, and Anne Magnus. 2011. The economic benefits of reducing physical inactivity: An Australian example. *International Journal of Behavioral Nutrition and Physical Activity* 8: 99. [CrossRef] [PubMed]

Dubey, Neha, Priyanka Podder, and Dinkar Pandey. 2020. Knowledge of COVID-19 and Its Influence on Mindfulness, Cognitive Emotion Regulation and Psychological Flexibility in the Indian Community. *Frontiers in Psychology* 11: 589365. [CrossRef] [PubMed]

Food and Health Bureau. 2021. The Government of the Hong Kong Special Administrative Region. Estimates of Health Expenditure: 1989/90–2019/20. Available online: https://www.fhb.gov.hk/statistics/en/dha/dha_summary_report.htm (accessed on 20 October 2021).

Greulich-Smith, Tamsin. 2020. Can Artificial Intelligence Care for the Elderly? Available online: https://govinsider.asia/smart-gov/ai-powering-dubais-pursuit-happiness/ (accessed on 24 October 2021).

Guure, Chris B., Noor A. Ibrahim, Mohd B. Adam, and Salmiah Md Said. 2017. Impact of Physical Activity on Cognitive Decline, Dementia, and Its Subtypes: Meta-Analysis of Prospective Studies. *BioMed Research International* 2017: 9016924. [CrossRef] [PubMed]

Hafner, Marco, Erez Yerushalmi, William D. Phillips, Jack Pollard, Advait Deshpande, Michael Whitmore, Francois Millard, and Christian Van Stolk. 2019. *The Economic Benefits of a More Physically Active Population: An International Analysis.* Santa Monica: RAND Corporation, RR-4291-TVG. Available online: https://www.rand.org/pubs/research_reports/RR4291.html (accessed on 14 January 2022).

Hafner, Marco, Erez Yerushalmi, Martin Stepanek, William Phillips, Jack Pollard, Advait Deshpande, Michael Whitmore, Francois Millard, Shaun Subel, and Christian Van Stolk. 2020. Estimating the global economic benefits of physically active populations over 30 years (2020–2050). *British Journal of Sports Medicine* 54: 1482–87. [CrossRef] [PubMed]

Hupin, David, Frédéric Roche, Vincent Gremeaux, Jean-Claude Chatard, Mathieu Oriol, Jean-Michel Gaspoz, Jean-Claude Barthélémy, and Pascal Edouard. 2015. Even a low-dose of moderate-to-vigorous physical activity reduces mortality by 22% in adults aged≥60 years: A systematic review and meta-analysis. *British Journal of Sports Medicine* 49: 1262–67. [CrossRef] [PubMed]

Marashi, Maryam Yvonne, Emma Nicholson, Michelle Ogrodnik, Barbara Fenesi, and Jennifer J. Heisz. 2021. A mental health paradox: Mental health was both a motivator and barrier to physical activity during the COVID-19 pandemic. *PLoS ONE* 16: e0239244. [CrossRef] [PubMed]

Nilsen, Per, Ida Seing, Carin Ericsson, Ove Andersen, Nina Thórný Stefánsdóttir, Tine Tjørnhøj-Thomsen, Thomas Kallemose, and Jeanette Wassar Kirk. 2020. Implementing social distancing policy measures in the battle against the coronavirus: Protocol of a comparative study of Denmark and Sweden. *Implementation Science Communications* 1: 77. [CrossRef] [PubMed]

Portegijs, Erja, Kirsi E. Keskinen, Johanna Eronen, Milla Saajanaho, Merja Rantakokko, and Taina Rantanen. 2020. Older Adults' Physical Activity and the Relevance of Distances to Neighborhood Destinations and Barriers to Outdoor Mobility. *Frontiers in Public Health* 8: 335. [CrossRef] [PubMed]

Portegijs, Erja, Kirsi E. Keskinen, Essi-Mari Tuomola, Timo Hinrichs, Milla Saajanaho, and Taina Rantanen. 2021. Older adults' activity destinations before and during COVID-19 restrictions: From a variety of activities to mostly physical exercise close to home. *Health Place* 68: 102533. [CrossRef] [PubMed]

Schuch, Felipe B., Davy Vancampfort, Joseph Firth, Simon Rosenbaum, Philip B. Ward, Edson S. Silva, Mats Hallgren, Antonio Ponce De Leon, Andrea L. Dunn, Andrea C. Deslandes, and et al. 2018. Physical Activity and Incident Depression: A Meta-Analysis of Prospective Cohort Studies. *American Journal of Psychiatry* 175: 631–48. [CrossRef] [PubMed]

Shah, Tejal M., Michael Weinborn, Giuseppe Verdile, Hamid R. Sohrabi, and Ralph N. Martins. 2017. Enhancing Cognitive Functioning in Healthly Older Adults: A Systematic Review of the Clinical Significance of Commercially Available Computerized Cognitive Training in Preventing Cognitive Decline. *Neuropsychology Review* 27: 62–80. [CrossRef] [PubMed]

Stay Physically Active during Self-Quarantine. 2020. WHO. Available online: https://www.euro.who.int/en/health-topics/health-emergencies/coronavirus-covid-19/technical-guidance/stay-physically-active-during-self-quarantine (accessed on 22 October 2021).

Stephenson, John, Bauman Adrian, Armstrong Tim, Smith Ben, and Bellew Bill. 2000. The Cost of Illness Attributable to Physical Inactivity in Australia; A Preliminary Study. Available online: https://www1.health.gov.au/internet/main/publishing.nsf/Content/5F2C0F157D587DAECA257BF0001E44CE/$File/phys_costofillness.pdf (accessed on 20 October 2021).

Suzuki, Yuta, Noriaki Maeda, Daigo Hirado, Taizan Shirakawa, and Yukio Urabe. 2020. Physical Activity Changes and Its Risk Factors among Community-Dwelling Japanese Older Adults during the COVID-19 Epidemic: Associations with Subjective Well-Being and Health-Related Quality of Life. *International Journal of Environmental Research and Public Health* 17: 6591. [CrossRef]

Tak, Erwin, Rebecca Kuiper, Astrid Chorus, and Marijke Hopman-Rock. 2013. Prevention of onset and progression of basic ADL disability by physical activity in community dwelling older adults: A meta-analysis. *Ageing Research Reviews* 12: 329–38. [CrossRef] [PubMed]

The Best Health and Fitness Apps for Seniors. 2020. Available online: https://www.thetechhelper.com/health-fitness-apps-seniors/ (accessed on 20 October 2021).

Watson, Kathleen B., Susan A. Carlson, Janelle P. Gunn, Deborah A. Galuska, Ann O'Connor, Kurt J. Greenlund, and Janet E. Fulton. 2016. Physical Inactivity Among Adults Aged 50 Years and Older—United States, 2014. *MMWR. Morbidity and Mortality Weekly Report* 65: 954–58. [CrossRef]

Yamada, Minoru, Yasuyuki Kimura, Daisuke Ishiyama, Yuhei Otobe, Mizue Suzuki, Shingo Koyama, Takashi Kikuchi, Hitomi Kusumi, and Hajime Arai. 2020. Effect of the COVID-19 Epidemic on Physical Activity in Community-Dwelling Older Adults in Japan: A Cross-Sectional Online Survey. *The Journal of Nutrition, Health & Aging* 24: 948–50. [CrossRef]

Zbrońska, Izabela, and Ewa Mędrela-Kuder. 2018. The level of physical activity in elderly persons with overweight and obesity. *Roczniki Państwowego Zakładu Higieny* 69: 369–73. [CrossRef]

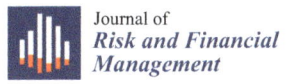

Editorial

COVID-19: An Economic or Social Disease? Implications for Disadvantaged Populations

Hijrah Nasir [1], **Valentin Navel** [2], **Julien S Baker** [3], **Rashmi Supriya** [3,*], **Alistair Cole** [4], **Yang Gao** [3] **and Frederic Dutheil** [5]

[1] Economic Development, Université Clermont Auvergne, F-63000 Clermont-Ferrand, France; hijrahnasir2013@gmail.com
[2] Université Clermont Auvergne, CNRS, INSERM, GReD, Translational Approach to Epithelial Injury and Repair, CHU Clermont-Ferrand, University Hospital of Clermont-Ferrand, Ophthalmology, F-63000 Clermont-Ferrand, France; valentin.navel@hotmail.fr
[3] Centre for Health and Exercise Science Research, Department of Sport, Physical Education and Health, Hong Kong Baptist University, Kowloon Tong 999077, Hong Kong; jsbaker@hkbu.edu.hk (J.S.B.); gaoyang@hkbu.edu.hk (Y.G.)
[4] Department of Government and International Studies, Hong Kong Baptist University, Kowloon Tong 999077, Hong Kong; alistaircole@hkbu.edu.hk
[5] Université Clermont Auvergne, CNRS, LaPSCo, Physiological and Psychosocial Stress, CHU Clermont-Ferrand, University Hospital of Clermont-Ferrand, Preventive and Occupational Medicine, Witty Fit, F-63000 Clermont-Ferrand, France; fdutheil@chu-clermontferrand.fr
* Correspondence: Rashmisupriya@hkbu.edu.hk

Citation: Nasir, Hijrah, Valentin Navel, Julien S Baker, Rashmi Supriya, Alistair Cole, Yang Gao, and Frederic Dutheil. 2021. COVID-19: An Economic or Social Disease? Implications for Disadvantaged Populations. *Journal of Risk and Financial Management* 14: 587. https://doi.org/10.3390/jrfm14120587

Academic Editor: Thanasis Stengos

Received: 17 November 2021
Accepted: 30 November 2021
Published: 6 December 2021

Publisher's Note: MDPI stays neutral with regard to jurisdictional claims in published maps and institutional affiliations.

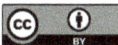

Copyright: © 2021 by the authors. Licensee MDPI, Basel, Switzerland. This article is an open access article distributed under the terms and conditions of the Creative Commons Attribution (CC BY) license (https://creativecommons.org/licenses/by/4.0/).

The world is still struggling against the coronavirus (COVID-19) pandemic. Inclusive of November 2021, the virus has already caused the death of more than 5.1 million people globally (WHO 2021). This pandemic brings many additional consequences, including economic and social instability. The economic implications are detrimental not only to public health systems but also to trade and travel, the food and agriculture industries, various market traders, and retail chains, among others (Evans 2020). The lockdown regulations imposed by governments in many countries decreased productivity in industry and food consumption rates. Accordingly, the annual global Gross Domestic Product growth was projected to drop to 2.4% in 2020, from an already weak 2.9% in 2019, with negative growth being predicted in the first quarter of 2021 (OECD Interim Economic Assessment 2020). The implications of the pandemic have been outlined as the worst global financial decline since the Great Depression of the 1930s. This situation has worsened in developing countries. For instance, the economic growth in the Sub-Saharan Africa region plunged to −2.1% and decreased to a record low of −5.1% in 2021 due to the COVID-19 global crisis (The World Bank 2020). This was partly due to a sharp decline in output growth of consumer partners and a severe drop in oil prices. As a result, recent research has predicted that economic contraction caused by COVID-19 could push an additional 500 million people (about 8 percent of the Earth's population) into poverty, reversing 30 years of economic development (Turse 2020) As increasing numbers of workers become unemployed as a direct result of the virus, it appears that the virus is not only causing severe illness and death, but also perpetuating a decline in economic conditions among poor people (Crayne 2020). Not surprisingly, negative economic implications are followed by social problems in many countries around the world. Xenophobia and racism related to the coronavirus pandemic have reportedly increased both offline and on social media. Physical attacks against Chinese and other Asian people, increased hate propaganda and speeches blaming Roma and Hispanic people for the spread of the virus, and calls by some political leaders for migrants to be denied access to medical services have been reported around the world since the start of the outbreak (United Nation News 2020; Cheng 2020).

Lockdown, confinement, and quarantine coupled with deteriorating socioeconomic conditions have significantly increased the risk of intimate partner violence. In Argentina,

Canada, France, Germany, Spain, the United Kingdom, and the United States, government authorities, women's rights activists, and civil society partners have highlighted increasing reports of domestic violence during the crisis and the heightened demand for emergency shelter for vulnerable individuals (Mlambo-Ngcuka 2020; Roesch et al. 2020). It has also been reported that certain sections of the population resorted to panic-buying in the shops and supermarkets with a significant surge in demand to purchase large quantities of consumables in anticipation of being at home for long periods of time (Yuen et al. 2020). This caused merchandise and food shortages for retailers around the world, especially for face masks, hand sanitizer, and some basic supplies such as noodles, rice, and toilet paper (Wu et al. 2020). During the pandemic, governments in many countries have enforced lockdowns or confinement, which have led to a decrease in social interaction between individuals and families. As a result of social distancing, the interaction between families and friends has been limited. This lack of social interaction may increase susceptibility to stress, anxiety, and depression (Park et al. 2020). Governments and policy makers perpetuate the health concept as a "physical health parameter", while mental wellness and a stable mental condition have, unfortunately, been secondary concerns.

There are staggering economic costs associated with social distancing. Many people find social distancing frustrating, but the economic repercussions of distancing are devastating to the most vulnerable, poorest, and marginalized members of our society. There are trade-offs that do not seem to have been adequately considered, even when considering lives lost, injuries sustained, and lifelong psychological damage. A high unemployment rate may result in higher levels of suicide, substance abuse, domestic violence, poverty, homelessness, and hunger. As a result of individuals feeling frustrated and having to stay at home in isolation for longer periods than normal, frustration, bad temper, and bouts of anxiety may occur. This could result in increased incidence of domestic violence occurring more regularly (Stefanie DeLuca 2021).

A further concern is that social distancing or long-term quarantine measures may not be sustainable when there is a wide disparity between the disadvantaged sections of the population and the more advantaged. Further to this, it is also clear that business as usual has intolerable consequences. However, when social and economic costs are acknowledged, they are usually treated as footnotes rather than as priorities. Social distancing appears to be a case of a "cost–benefit" analysis, regardless of whether we agree with it or not. Shuttering the economy permanently is unsustainable because those bearing the greatest financial burdens are unlikely to comply with social distancing rules.

Sociologists have tried to examine what motivates people to take risks or avoid risks in general. During the pandemic, it is not feasible to ask the marginalized among us to sit through weeks or months of social distancing. Creating policies that assume that families with no food to eat will remain at home for long periods is a mistake. Several of these factors have led to social problems and contributed to psychological problems in society as a result of the pandemic. It becomes increasingly difficult to recover from aggregate economic effects with increasing time. In addition, as each day passes, the burden on families increases. The longer the pandemic continues, the less likely it is that the individuals feeling the greatest financial implications of social isolation will follow public health guidance. Sections of society cannot be expected to make such sacrifices, in relation to financial constraints and sustainability. In order to understand basic information such as infection and mortality rates, it is imperative that we begin testing systematically sampled subsets of the population. In relation to the current status of the global COVID-19 pandemic, efforts to stem the pandemic are stymied by the lack of reliable information or the difficulty of interpreting collected data. COVID-19 treatment strategies and management of the pandemic may eventually lead to more targeted interventions with less economic impact when transmission, infection rates, and COVID-19 management strategies are better understood. Rather than coping with the spread of the virus rationally, we are compelled to implement radical, blanket measures that impose staggering costs on vulnerable subsets of the population.

Research is needed in order to avoid this disorganized, deadly response occurring again in the future. There is also a need to revisit policy changes and legislative government policy implementation to provide viable alternative responses to the pandemic. The pandemic will have direct health consequences for the medical profession and infected individuals, but as a society, we must also learn lessons about the costs, sacrifice, and human behavior responses to such an event. This includes physiological, psychological, and medical consequences and encompasses issues such as what groups of individuals are willing to help, are able to cope, or will suffer pandemic consequences. It would be prudent to examine the relative effectiveness of our current social safety net. This would include an examination of what policies have proven to be the most effective and what policies and strategies have been least successful. Traditional antipoverty programs cannot be used when there is social distancing. When people with resources buy in bulk, they purchase the food that low-income parents need, thus negating the purpose of Electronic Benefit Transfer benefits. When landlords cannot meet with inspectors or prospective tenants as part of the leasing process, housing vouchers are less likely to lessen housing burdens. Without technology, it is impossible to provide certain special education services outside the classroom and at home. It is crucial that we pay attention to those intermediaries who have contributed to reducing costs, such as teachers and social workers who have risked their own health to provide therapy and assistance to the poorest families. We have both an opportunity and a responsibility to improve our support services not only for the next pandemic, but for every pandemic in the future. Now is the time to learn lessons and make important changes that will assist in creating realistic, implementable, supportive, and effective governmental policies in the future.

Author Contributions: H.N., V.N., F.D., J.S.B. and R.S. wrote the paper. A.C. and Y.G. contributed to discussion and editing. All authors have read and agreed to the published version of the manuscript.

Funding: This research received no external funding.

Institutional Review Board Statement: Not applicable.

Informed Consent Statement: Not applicable.

Data Availability Statement: Not applicable.

Acknowledgments: This paper was prepared from a presentation on this idea, presented in the symposium "Transnational and Transdisciplinary Lessons of COVID-19 from the Perspective of Risk and Management".

Conflicts of Interest: The authors declare no conflict of interest.

References

Cheng, Shuliang Oliver. 2020. Xenophobia due to the coronavirus outbreak—A letter to the editor in response to "the socio-economic implications of the coronavirus pandemic (COVID-19): A review". *International Journal of Surgery* 79: 13–14. [CrossRef] [PubMed]

Crayne, Matthew P. 2020. The traumatic impact of job loss and job search in the aftermath of covid-19. *Psychological Trauma: Theory, Research, Practice, and Policy* 12: s180–s182. [CrossRef]

Evans, Olaniyi. 2020. Socio-Economic Impacts of Novel Coronavirus: The Policy Solutions. Econpapers. Available online: https://econpapers.repec.org/article/risbuecqu/0013.htm (accessed on 10 November 2021).

Mlambo-Ngcuka, Phumzile. 2020. Violence against Women and Girls: The Shadow Pandemic. UN Women. Available online: https://www.unwomen.org/en/news/stories/2020/4/statement-ed-phumzile-violence-against-women-during-pandemic#notes (accessed on 10 November 2021).

OECD Interim Economic Assessment. 2020. Coronavirus: The World Economy at Risk. Available online: https://www.oecd.org/berlin/publikationen/interim-economic-assessment-2-march-2020.pdf (accessed on 10 November 2021).

Park, Crystal L., Beth S. Russell, Michael Fendrich, Lucy Finkelstein-Fox, Morica Hutchison, and Jessica Becker. 2020. Americans' COVID-19 stress, coping, and adherence to cdc guidelines. *Journal of General Internal Medicine* 35: 2296–303. [CrossRef]

Roesch, Elisabeth, Avni Amin, Jhumka Gupta, and Claudia García-Moreno. 2020. Violence against women during covid-19 pandemic restrictions. *BMJ*, m1712. [CrossRef] [PubMed]

Stefanie DeLuca, James Coleman. 2021. The Unequal Cost of Social Distancing. OHNS Hopkins University & Medicine. Available online: https://coronavirus.jhu.edu/from-our-experts/the-unequal-cost-of-social-distancing (accessed on 27 October 2021).

The World Bank. 2020. COVID-19 (Coronavirus) Drives Sub-Saharan Africa toward First Recession in 25 Years. Available online: https://www.worldbank.org/en/news/press-release/2020/04/09/covid-19-coronavirus-drives-sub-saharan-africa-toward-first-recession-in-25-years (accessed on 10 November 2021).

Turse, Nick. 2020. Exceptionally Dire: Secondary Impacts of COVID-19 Could Increase Global Poverty and Hunger. The Intercept. Available online: https://theintercept.com/2020/05/03/exceptionally-dire-secondary-impacts-of-covid-19-could-increase-global-poverty-and-hunger/ (accessed on 10 November 2021).

United Nation News. 2020. COVID-19 Stoking Xenophobia, Hate and Exclusion, Minority Rights Expert Warns. Available online: https://news.un.org/en/story/2020/03/1060602 (accessed on 10 November 2021).

WHO. 2021. Who Coronavirus (COVID-19) Dashboard. Available online: https://covid19.who.int/ (accessed on 16 November 2021).

Wu, Huai-liang, Jian Huang, Casper Zhang, Zonglin He, and Wai-Kit Minga. 2020. Facemask shortage and the novel coronavirus disease (covid-19) outbreak: Reflections on public health measures. *Eclinicalmedicine* 21: 100329. [CrossRef] [PubMed]

Yuen, Kum Fai, Xueqin Wang, Fei Ma, and Kevin X. Li. 2020. The psychological causes of panic buying following a health crisis. *International Journal of Environmental Research And Public Health* 17: 3513. [CrossRef] [PubMed]

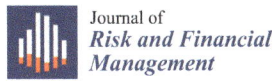

Article

Trust, Transparency and Welfare: Third-Sector Adult Social Care Delivery and the COVID-19 Pandemic in the UK

Paul Chaney * and Christala Sophocleous

Wales Institute of Social and Economic Research, Data and Methods (WISERD), Cardiff University, Cardiff CF10 3AT, UK; SophocleousC1@cardiff.ac.uk
* Correspondence: chaneyp@cardiff.ac.uk

Abstract: Since the move to quasi-federalism in the 1990s, different territorial welfare mixes on adult social care (ASC) have emerged in the four nations of the UK. This study explores policy actors' views on their effectiveness in the pandemic with reference to the role of institutions, trust and transparency. The analysis is based on extensive secondary data analysis and primary interviews with key individuals involved in the delivery and regulation of ASC. The findings highlight how the pandemic exposed existing pathologies and the need for reform in all four systems. Notably, the analysis shows how the present market-based tendering systems for allocating ASC contracts undermine inter-personal and institutional trust and compromise care quality. The wider significance of this lies in showing the pivotal role of trust during the emergency and that post-pandemic welfare reform needs to embed trust-building measures to deliver effective care.

Keywords: pandemic; social welfare; trust; transparency; adult social care; UK

Citation: Chaney, Paul, and Christala Sophocleous. 2021. Trust, Transparency and Welfare: Third-Sector Adult Social Care Delivery and the COVID-19 Pandemic in the UK. *Journal of Risk and Financial Management* 14: 572. https://doi.org/10.3390/jrfm14120572

Academic Editor: Julien S. Baker

Received: 7 October 2021
Accepted: 11 November 2021
Published: 26 November 2021

Publisher's Note: MDPI stays neutral with regard to jurisdictional claims in published maps and institutional affiliations.

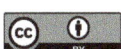

Copyright: © 2021 by the authors. Licensee MDPI, Basel, Switzerland. This article is an open access article distributed under the terms and conditions of the Creative Commons Attribution (CC BY) license (https:// creativecommons.org/licenses/by/ 4.0/).

1. Introduction

Since the move to quasi-federalism, different territorial welfare mixes on adult social care delivery have emerged in the four nations of the UK. This study compares policy actors' views on their effectiveness in adult social care (ASC) delivery during the pandemic with reference to the role of institutions, trust and transparency. The analysis is based on extensive secondary data analysis and primary interviews with key individuals involved in the delivery and regulation of ASC. The term 'adult social care' refers to non-medical support, including provision of social work, personal care, protection or social support services, to adults in need, typically arising from old age and/or disability. Specifically, we examine domiciliary care in the service user's home (not in residential care homes). By "welfare mixes", we refer to the mixed economy of welfare—or welfare pluralism. Typically, local government social services departments issue contracts to provide ASC to local communities. Government policy determines the prevailing welfare mix. Care providers are either in the state sector (employed by local government), work for private sector companies operating for profit, or belong to not-for-profit bodies in the third (or voluntary) sector. Definitions of the latter are contested (cf. Salamon and Anheier 1998). For the present purposes, the third sector denotes charities, NGOs and co-operatives. It is also sometimes referred to as the community sector. Such organisations may deliver ASC through voluntary activities and/or they may secure state funding to supplement their voluntary service provision with paid employees.

It is germane to consider why the issue of ASC is deserving of attention. The answer is a major increase in demand for care due to an international demographic shift towards an ageing population. In the UK, the number of people 65+ years is predicted to reach one-in-four people (24.2 per cent) by 2038 (ONS 2020). This global trend means we live in an era when, for first time in human history, the number of older people (60+ years) will exceed younger people. As a result of declining state capacity (owing to austerity, and latterly fiscal deficits incurred as part of the pandemic response), the UK Prime Minister has referred to a "crisis in social care". In consequence, third-sector adult care providers are increasingly in the front line of service providers for the vulnerable.

Against this backdrop, there is need for further scholarly work on the rise of mixed economies of welfare as a global phenomenon (Wigell 2017). Despite trust being a key variable in public support for state-organised welfare (Rose 1991; Rothstein 1998), to date, studies of social welfare have paid little attention to trust and multi-level governance (Daniele and Geys 2015). Moreover, the extant literature fails to take full account of how the mixed economy of welfare is grounded in the nature of political systems (Wigell 2017). In addition, classic welfare state theory (Esping-Andersen 1990; Arts and Gelissen 2002) tends to concentrate on state-wide practices, thereby overlooking the (increasing) significance of meso-level developments. As Daniele and Geys (2015, p. 3) observe, more work is needed on "the potential relevance for welfare state support of interpersonal trust among the members of a given community (over and above institutional trust)". While interpersonal trust has previously been linked to economic growth (Knack and Keefer 1997), financial development and international trade, its potential significance for welfare state support is limited. Dickinson et al. (2012, p. 24) concur: "Further research might also investigate the market niche that third-sector providers have in social care and examine how this is maintained, for example, through trust". There is also need for research on trust, welfare and inequalities. As Kevins (2019) underlines, the need to foster trust from welfare recipients that are labour-market outsiders (the majority of ASC users) is a particularly acute challenge as, typically, they exhibit lower levels of trust towards welfare providers.

Here, we engage with these lacunae and add to the current understanding of trust and the decentralization of the welfare state (Borghi and Van Berkel 2007; Chaney 2020a, 2020b). The present focus on meso-level developments is a corrective to the "methodological nationalism" of earlier state-wide research (Wimmer and Schiller 2002). It reflects the fact that the nature of prevailing welfare mixes is grounded in territorial electoral politics and political ideology (Chaney 2021). This matters because, as Henderson et al. (2013, p. 146) note, "[citizens] usually have more trust in regional than in national institutions". Today's quasi-federal UK can be viewed as a natural experiment in this regard. Lastly, whilst there is a literature on welfare delivery in the context of major emergencies, this is largely restricted to development studies. Here, we seek to extend this to consider the impact of the pandemic on ASC following the UK's move to multi-level governance.

The remainder of this paper is structured as follows. Following an outline of the study methodology, the findings are presented. These consider each territory in turn. First, the nature of the mixed economy model of ASC applying in each is outlined ("Research Context"), followed by examination of policy actors' views on the extent to which the four mixed economy models provided an effective response to ASC delivery in the pandemic, with reference to the role of trust and transparency ("Research Findings"). The discussion and conclusion reflect on the study findings and their implications.

2. Methods

This is a mixed methods study involving primary and secondary data analysis. In social theory terms, it uses qualitative discourse analysis because, as the interpretive school of policy analysis and social constructivism (Kukla 2000) underline, social research benefits from emphasis on values, beliefs, narratives and interpretations germane to a given policy issue (Eden and Ackermann 2004). Thus, it eschews quantification of interview responses and instead embraces standpoint theory. This is suited to exploring the "situated knowledge" (Stoetzler and Yuval-Davis 2002) of policy actors in relation to the delivery of social care before and during the pandemic. In this regard, it is methodologically concerned with the inherent meanings, messages and criticality in relation to social experience (Druckman 2001). It is allied to the classic work of Goffman (1974) and discursive framing or the language used by policy actors and the inherent meanings, sentiments, emotions, messages and criticality in relation to social and political communication (Heine and Narrog 2015).

The primary data analysis comprised a sample of a hundred interviews with civil society policy actors and other stakeholders undertaken prior to, and during, the pandemic, 2017–2021. Purposive sampling was used to achieve a spread of interviewees, with a target of approximately 25 in each of the four nations (Godwill 2015; Campbell et al. 2020; Stratton 2021). The constraints of lockdown during the COVID-19 pandemic meant that the methodology was adapted from pre-COVID face-to-face data-gathering to online interviews during lockdown (via Zoom and similar digital platforms). The term "policy actors" here refers to those working for: third-sector organizations (TSOs) delivering domiciliary social care; bodies representing TSOs on regional partnership forums and other governance settings; and statutory commissions and inspectorates concerned with care standards, equality and human rights. The interviews that we secured were recorded and professionally transcribed. The transcripts were manually coded using deductive coding to identify emerging themes (Fereday and Muir-Cochrane 2006). As the burgeoning research methods literature attests (MacPhail et al. 2015; Saldaña 2021), manual coding was selected in preference to analytical software because it allows the researcher greater immersion in the dataset (Basit 2003; James 2013) and is often more accurate in understanding colloquial language use, as well as ambiguities, speaker emphasis and use of rhetorical devices, including irony (Mattimoe et al. 2021).

Following established methodological practice (see Natow 2020), the interview findings were triangulated with document analysis (Bowen 2009). The secondary data analysis involved exhaustive online keyword searches of parliamentary websites and those of CSOs and statutory regulators of ASC in the UK. Purposive sampling was again used to achieve documentary coverage across the four nations of the UK (Godwill 2015; Campbell et al. 2020). This rich dataset included extensive evidence submitted to a series of parliamentary inquiries on the response to the COVID-19 pandemic, such as the UK Parliament's Select Committee on Culture, Media and Sport inquiry on the impact of COVID-19 on the charity sector. Again, electronic versions of these documents were manually coded for emerging themes using Adobe Acrobat or the annotation tool for webpages in the Microsoft Edge web-browser (Mackieson et al. 2019).

3. Research Context

In this section, we succinctly outline the nature of the mixed economy model of ASC applying in each territory.

3.1. Wales

The Welsh mixed economy model of social care delivery is distinctive. Under Welsh law, specifically, the Social Services and Well-being (Wales) Act, 2014, local (or municipal) government is placed under a statutory duty to promote third-sector organisations' delivery of social care. From the outset, third-sector policy actors have highlighted the pivotal role of trust in their working with government. As one observed, "It wouldn't function without trust ... hard won, easily lost, isn't it?—trust". Despite the collectivist political aspiration of successive socialist/civic nationalist governments in Wales, a marketised, private sector dominated system endures. Two-thirds of ASC staff are in the in private (or "for profit") sector. The third and public sectors each employ 17 per cent of the ASC workforce (IFC Consulting 2018). This is unsurprising, as prior to devolution in 1999 Wales and England largely shared the same legal and policy framework (and, as we shall see below, English policy promoted private sector welfare delivery). Third-sector interviewees in the present study lauded the legislative approach of promoting third-sector ASC. However, they were also critical of 2014 Act. Far from promoting collectivism, they highlighted how it has led to marketisation and reinforced inequalities—not least, because of the "widespread use of spot contracts and brokerage systems" (Atkinson et al. 2016, p. 2). Policy actors refer to how these cause instability and uncertainty about third-sector ASC organisations' long-term survival.

3.2. Scotland

A mixed-economy, marketised system of ASC operates in Scotland. Half of ASC staff are employed by third-sector organisations (the highest proportion in the UK). The remainder are in the public (23 per cent) and private sectors (31 per cent) (ICF 2018c). The current Scottish mixed economy model of ASC provision is set out in a complex raft of enactments that policy actors say tends to undermine transparency. Notably, the Community Care and Health (Scotland) Act 2002 introduced the totemic policy of "free" personal care for adults, regardless of income or whether they live at home or in residential care (in contrast to Wales and England where ASC is means-tested, and many have to pay for care). When related to the wider welfare literature, earlier work (e.g., Uslaner 2002) suggests that universal programmes might "increase trust by enhancing equality, optimism and the perception of individual opportunity" (Kevins 2019, p. 877). However, in part, the present findings contradict this premise. Policy actors were critical of several aspects of Scotland's mixed economy model. As Cunningham et al. (2019, p. 17) note, the Self-Directed Support (Scotland) Act (2013) (Scottish Parliament 2013) has promoted the marketization of care that has proved highly problematic for third-sector ASC providers. Many are critical of the commodification of ASC and the dehumanising language associated with it. One noted that, "We have reached a point where the commodification has in effect become the service. We have opted to put those services in place through a market mechanism which describes people's care and support arrangements as "packages"; we divide groups of people with support needs into "client groups" and bundle them into "lots", to be tendered on the market" (Coalition of Care and Support Providers in Scotland 2020, p. 3).

3.3. Northern Ireland

Northern Ireland also has a marketised system. Almost half of ASC workers are employed in the private sector. The public sector accounts for 30.1 per cent and the third-sector 23 per cent (ICF 2018b). From an institutional perspective, the province of Northern Ireland is different to the other countries in the UK because social care is integrated into the public healthcare system. In common with Scotland, Northern Ireland has free-at-the-point-of-delivery entitlement to personal care for adults regardless of income or whether they live at home or in residential care settings.

3.4. England

The nature of the mixed economy model of ASC in England is distinctive because of its neo-liberal approach. This is politically motivated—shaped by successive right-of-centre governments that eschew state provision and embrace contracting out to the private sector. In turn, this is reflected in the composition of the ASC workforce. Two-thirds of staff are employed in the private sector (64.8 per cent); just under a third are in the voluntary sector (31.9 per cent), whilst the public sector accounts for just 3.3 per cent (ICF 2018a). A recent review gave a withering critique of systemic ASC failings in England: "Short-term funding and the lack of a long-term vision has hampered planning, innovation and investment in adult social care. The current accountability and oversight arrangements are ineffective for overseeing the care market" (National Audit Office 2021, p. 6). Another concluded that major challenges stem from the complex and fragmented nature of the current system (Care Quality Commission 2019).

4. Research Findings

This section is structured to consider each territory in turn and examine policy actors' views on the response to ASC delivery in the pandemic.

4.1. Wales

The Welsh Government's pandemic response for third-sector ASC provision was included in a comprehensive emergency funding package for the sector as a whole. The official response also saw the relaxing of some bureaucratic rules on third-sector funding and service delivery. A key example of the emergency funding measures was the Third-Sector Resilience Fund, a blended loan and grant scheme designed to help third-sector organisations (TSOs) pay their bills and ease their cash-flow. Another was the Voluntary Services Emergency Fund, intended to enable more people to volunteer during the pandemic by coordinating the volunteer response and paying volunteers' out of pocket expenses.

The move to devolved government for Wales in the 1990s saw partnership working between government and third-sector embedded in constitutional law. During the pandemic, a government minister described this infrastructure as being "a huge positive". Policy actors also spoke of how, "successive Welsh Governments have invested in the third-sector and supported mechanisms for joint-working. It is notable that through the pandemic [. . . it] has continued to work through these existing structures, strengthening but not replacing them" (Welsh Parliament/Senedd Cymru 2021, p. 11). Third-sector policy actors also underlined the importance of the interpersonal and institutional trust built up through an extended history of working with meso-government. For example, one said: "for us that trust is a key thing. We have a lot of trust in the . . . [Welsh Government] officials that we work with, because some of those relationships are going back a decade. So, each time you take on a new area of policy or new bit of work, we have to work a little bit less hard to establish trust". Policy actors also referred to how, "the voluntary sector played an invaluable role in sharing essential messages to communities and the people they support, particularly at the outset of the pandemic" (Welsh Parliament/Senedd Cymru 2021, para 47). Interviewees also spoke of how the third-sector provided local care (foodbanks, community transport, etc.) when state ASC provision was compromised by staff contracting COVID-19 and being hospitalised or self-isolating. The pandemic also saw a dramatic surge in volunteers keen to help in the emergency. However, reflecting wider international experience (Asmorowati et al. 2021), study participants highlight how a major shortcoming was the poor level of strategic co-ordination of volunteers. Policy actors also referred to the compounding of difficulties experienced during the pandemic because it coincided with a number of ongoing reform agendas, including health service reorganization and Brexit (many ASC providers lost employees as a result of Brexit, most noticeably from Eastern European counties). Notwithstanding these challenges, third-sector policy actors confirmed that, in the words of one, "a combination of the funding available from various governments has meant that many voluntary sector organisations have been able to 'weather the storm'".

4.2. Scotland

One of the principal elements in the Scottish Government's pandemic response was a £350 million ($484 million) fund to support the welfare and wellbeing of those most affected by the coronavirus pandemic. This was open to local government, charities, businesses and community groups. Its aim was to "be focused on delivery, not bureaucracy or red tape". In consequence one policy actor reflected, "There has been more trust and less emphasis on reporting and monitoring, and we would really like that to continue". During the pandemic, additional funding was also added to the Scottish Welfare Fund (which makes community and crisis grants available to those in immediate need), the Food Fund (to help voluntary sector organisations address issues of food insecurity, especially for older people) and Wellbeing Fund (to help charities and others who require additional capacity to work with at-risk people who may be worst affected by the crisis).

In the wake of the pandemic, one third-sector leader reflected that, "Reform of social care in Scotland is long overdue. The COVID-19 pandemic has exposed fault lines which require radical overhaul and long-term change. It has also revealed what can be achieved when obstacles are removed in a crisis". Another questioned, "Can we use hard lessons learnt during COVID-19 to value social care more, and find new ways of supporting and valuing our most vulnerable citizens?" (SCVO 2020a, p. 5). Others referred to what they saw as problematic eligibility rules for the emergency aid. In particular, they complained that, under charities law, third-sector organisations relying on their reserves were not eligible for immediate crisis funding. They were only eligible when their funds were exhausted—effectively when they failed financially.

A common trope amongst policy actors was how the pandemic will drive future reform. For example, one parliamentarian said:

> We must embrace the adversity of the pandemic and seize it as an opportunity to do things differently. We must learn from innovative practice shown by some funders and the third sector during the pandemic. The COVID crisis has shone a light on the issues impacting the sector and on inequality in our society.

Throughout, trust was a consistent theme. Notably, the Scottish Parliament's Report on the impact of the COVID-19 pandemic on equalities and human rights underlined the need for, "greater transparency and scrutiny of the changes to social care, including information on the criteria and tools used by public bodies in their decision-making, and what measures are being taken to ensure ongoing monitoring" (SPEHRC 2021, p. 28). Whilst the representative body of the third sector said: "the pandemic has exacerbated inequalities ... Confidence in voluntary sector services exists because of the work to nurture trusting relationships between the organisations and the people they work with. This allows the sector to gather lived experience to advocate for change, and these relationships also make the sector well-placed to work with those most disengaged and isolated" (SCVO 2020b, p. 10, para 53).

4.3. Northern Ireland

Policy actors are highly critical of the current situation in Northern Ireland. As one noted, "fundamental reform of adult care and support is required to avoid a total collapse of the system with all the implications this would have for those in need. This requires both leadership and ownership across the whole system of care and support". A key issue is that, in the words of one TSO manager, "the current mechanisms have not been successful in creating or enabling a mixed economy of service provision". A major failing is the way that the independent social care sector is struggling to recruit and retain staff. This is due to the low pay that ASC workers receive, with many leaving to take up posts in the hospitality and retail sectors of the economy. Whilst these typically offer low pay, it is often more than remuneration in social care. According to stakeholders, this is creating the "perfect storm" because it is combining with the negative effects of Brexit, austerity and decades of inequality and poverty.

Despite these difficulties, policy actors praised the response of third-sector ASC providers during the pandemic. As one put it, "the community sector came to the fore in ways that other sectors couldn't and wouldn't and I think the status of the community sector has been enhanced considerably ... they naturally stood up to the plate when lockdown came in and services were required. I mean, half, if not three-quarters of the public sector was at home" (i.e., incapacitated by COVID). They also highlighted the beneficial effects of government suspension of bureaucracy and red tape during the crisis. For example, one noted: "there was definitely an instant flexibility and rolling forward of funding arrangements for the next 12 months—you know, without too much scrutiny".

Reflecting on the impact of the pandemic on ASC, a government minister said: "it is important to continue this new way of working after Covid-19. Against the backdrop of a society that is facing increasing pressures compounded by the uncertainties presented of Brexit, a restrictive overall budget, decades of inequality and poverty, and poor mental health, it is important to continue the collaborative way of working demonstrated over the last few months". She proceeded to describe "three key pillars" under which she believes the current work can continue: partnership and collaboration, co-design and co-production, and delivery of real improvements and real outcomes. Yet, when responding to the Northern Ireland Executive's pandemic recovery plan, third-sector policy actors said that the government needed to do more to address economic inequality and promote human rights in ASC (Northern Ireland Executive Department for Health 2020, pp. 9–12).

4.4. England

The English pandemic response consisted of £750 million ($1 billion) of financial support for voluntary, community and social enterprises, including those delivering ASC. During the COVID emergency, a thousand third-sector organisations were surveyed by government. This revealed that almost half had accessed the government support packages. However, when asked about the effectiveness of the aid, almost half of respondents (43 per cent) gave negative replies (Department for Digital, Culture, Media and Sport and Office for Civil Society 2021). One TSO explained, "the Covid-19 crisis ... may tip over the charity. We are fighting hard to avoid this outcome [... we have suffered a] Loss of 70 per cent of our volunteers who are now self-isolating; and a loss of 90 per cent of our income over night".

Equalities and human rights organisations raised several concerns about the government's COVID response: "the government and public services must not use any new powers to undermine people's human rights and rights to equality and non-discrimination. The powers must be used in ways that are non-discriminatory and proportionate to achieving the legitimate aim of responding to the epidemic". The national representative body for third-sector organisations in England warned: "Charities across the country are facing imminent collapse as fundraising income dries up ... Community and voluntary sector organisations are also on the frontline of supporting vulnerable people and will experience a variety of impacts related to the crisis. Some are seeing huge increases in demand for services". For many care providers, survival was the key issue. One observed, "The crisis is biting us hard. Even with us doing everything we can (such as furloughing staff, applying for business support, paid staff voluntarily cutting their wages etc.). We will not be able to continue beyond the next few months if nothing substantial changes".

Others spoke of how, in their view, the pandemic response was compounding inequalities: "There is currently no clarity on what, if any, consideration will be given to equality and equity, including the need to fund organisations that represent marginalised communities. Poorer areas of the country ... feel the impacts of a reduction in services far more than wealthier parts of the country". This TSO concluded: "put simply, the government's intervention will not be enough to prevent good charities around the country from closing their doors. Many of the charities which do survive will look very different in a few months' time, with severely reduced capacity to provide support that people rely on at a time when their contribution to recovery will be vital".

(Mis)trust was a key issue in the marginalisation and inequalities experienced by black and minority ethnic (BAME) communities in England during the pandemic. Thus, a report by the state healthcare regulator called for improved access, experiences and outcomes of integrated care for black and minority ethnic communities. Recommended measures included, "integration of equality into quality systems; good representation of black and minority ethnic communities among staff at all levels [and] trust-building dialogue with service users" (Public Health England 2020, p. 10). Allied to this, one community leader told a government inquiry on the pandemic, "Muslim charities hold a great deal of trust with the communities they work with, but with rises in Islamophobia ... increased dialogue, communication and engagement with the Muslim charitable sector is recommended. During this unprecedented global crisis, it is imperative they are engaged with at the earliest possible time". Policy actors' discourse also reveals widespread anxiety that the organisations that support BAME groups may not survive due to the economic impact of the COVID-19 emergency. As one observer noted: "The prediction is that 40 per cent of SME community and voluntary sector will cease to exist in three months from now. Including those run by ethnic minorities supporting individuals with overlapping intersectionality (e.g., BAME, woman, single parent, mental illness, those not employed)—these small organisations will cease to exist ... my concern is that trust is diminished yet again for these communities—but how do we sustain and strengthen a sector that doesn't exist?" (Public Health England 2020, p. 28).

5. Discussion: The Pandemic and the Role of Trust and Transparency in the Mixed Economy of ASC Delivery

The current study reveals the pivotal role of trust in welfare delivery immediately prior to—and during, the pandemic. As one study participant noted "It's huge, isn't it? If you haven't got trust, you haven't got open dialogue, you haven't got interest or understanding of each other's positions". Trust was seen as vital to policy development and co-working with government. For example, one interviewee said, "I think there is quite a good amount of trust and respect for our organisation from ... government officials. And particularly with one particular person that we work with. And I think we're often seen as the 'go to' organisation for our knowledge and skills on particular subjects ... they value our opinion and our reputation. And I think that there's a lot of trust and respect there". Across the four territories, the current analysis shows the main (non-discrete) dimensions of trust are institutional (between institutions, and citizens' trust towards institutions); intra-institutional (e.g., ASC workers' trust towards the organisations they work for) and inter-personal (i.e., between individuals spanning organisational boundaries, and between welfare service users and providers). Trust is also integral to the future success of post-pandemic reforms, for as Habibov et al. (2019, p. 466) conclude: "welfare state reforms could prove be more effective within a social context where levels of trust are high. Thus, special attention should be paid to initiatives aimed at developing strategies to build trust".

In the case of institutional trust in the different territorial ASC systems in the UK, a key issue was how governance complexity undermines transparency and reduces trust on the part of third-sector organisations. As one interviewee put it "it's exposed more the need for trust and openness". A prime example is the complicated institutional structures associated with ASC delivery under the 2014 Act in Wales. This complexity has undermined the transparency of the system and, in turn, levels of third-sector trust in the new arrangements. The new institutional structures centre on Regional Partnership Boards (RPBs) designed to promote welfare pluralism and bring together state bodies, local government and the third-sector to meet the care and support needs of people in their area. In practice, the level of the third-sector's involvement in RPBs was found to be highly variable. In some areas, there was thorough-going engagement, yet in others non-engagement meant that third-sector organisations were effectively excluded from shaping local ASC delivery. In such instances, RPBs effectively became a 'rubber stamping' exercise. Reasons for third-sector organisations' non-engagement included uncertainty about different institutional remits in relation to ASC delivery and a lack of resources and capacity to engage with the broad range of implementation structures.

The current analysis reveals a broadly similar situation in Scotland. The representative body of the third-sector concluded: "People in Scotland have grown ever more critical of those with decision-making power. Trust between policymakers and the public has fallen and continues to do so. With this growing mistrust and cynicism comes the need to find ways of opening up decision-making processes throughout the country, making them accessible and transparent for all" (SCVO 2020a, p. 3). Policy actors' discourse refers to policy complexity undermining trust, transparency and accountability. In response, during the pandemic the Scottish Government announced a review of ASC provision. Its vision for the successor system underlines a mixed-economy approach whereby, "People organising and delivering social care work together [including ...] communities, community workers, mental health practitioners, GPs, nurses, hospitals, therapists, housing services, transport services, and others" (Scottish Government 2019, p. 14). The stated aim is for systems, processes and decision making where "the relationship between public, independent and third sector health and social care organisations is trusting and collaborative" (Scottish Government 2019, p. 14). The post-pandemic Independent Review of Social Care in Scotland also puts trust at the heart of its recommendations: "We also need a transformation of the way in which we plan, commission and procure social care support. We need an approach that builds trusting relationships rather than competition. We need to build partnerships not market-places" (Scottish Government 2021, p. 5).

As earlier work emphasises, the degree of institutional trust depends on the perceived ability of institutions to deliver the expected outcomes (Wong et al. 2011; Habibov et al. 2019). The current study highlights two dimensions to trust in the pandemic response: government officials' attitudes towards community groups and citizens' attitudes towards government (as well as state, private and third-sector ASC providers). In the former regard, our analysis shows the need for state bodies to exhibit greater levels of trust towards third-sector organisations. As extant work (Van de Walle and Lahat 2017, p. 1450) observes, "given the critical role of trust in the functioning of the welfare state ... further awareness and mechanisms for increasing the degree of trust of citizens among public officials are warranted". The current evidence reveals that officials' willingness to trust community groups was shaped by the effectiveness of the pandemic response. Thus, a Parliamentary inquiry heard that: "Practical cooperation at community level was often good with local authorities; though [officials'] willingness to trust community groups has been very mixed. Pre-existing relationships (which contributed to levels of trust) were a major predictor of close working links during Lockdown. However, the crisis did help breakdown some of the pre-crisis barriers to co-operation such as poor communication, risk aversion and silo working, as people in both the statutory and voluntary sectors were driven overwhelmingly by the crisis to do things differently" (Welsh Parliament 2021, p. 23). Professionalism was a key factor determining officials' level of trust in community ASC providers. As one interviewee noted: "I mean, I think there is an overarching thing that I feel sometimes in the third-sector—[namely,] that the statutory bodies don't trust us enough to be a professional organisation. They just think, they have a particular image of volunteers which doesn't relate to the truth so there is always this perception inequality about things". Existing work (e.g., Taylor-Gooby 2000) has also underlined the links between welfare, risk and trust. This was evident in the current study findings—notably, when interviewees alluded to the role of evidence in boosting trust. For example, one third-sector policy actor spoke of government officials seeking prior evidence before extending funding to community groups for service delivery: "we've also got a capital programme, which government started funding about ten years ago. That was all about trust—that was about us showing a local project that worked [before we were given funding]".

Across polities, institutional trust is a core trope in the discourse on post-pandemic ASC reforms. For example, one third-sector body referred to: "encouraging an ongoing changing of behaviours and culture to share power better locally, regionally and nationally [this] will, I think, build that greater resilience." Others talked of "hard-wiring" key relationships between different organisations where necessary and ensuring that decision makers "truly trust their colleagues in their communities ... ". Such measures "are essential ... hard-wiring relationships would build resilience and mean that there can be improved responses" (Welsh Parliament 2021, p. 43). Another interviewee put it simply, "the process and the infrastructure for those relationships is based around trust".

A further common theme was how inter-personal trust between policy actors increased the longer the duration of the working relationship. Familiarity was seen as key to interpersonal trust, and interviewees gave a number of examples of how and when staff left their posts and how this impacted on prevailing levels of trust and, in turn, the efficacy of the working relationship. For example, one noted that "we are finding increasingly that we're dealing with different people all the time, and that doesn't support us in building trust and building a common understanding, and a common appreciation of knowledge and skill base, really". The current findings also reveal how staff retention issues during the pandemic negatively impacted on inter-personal trust between third-sector service care providers and service users. Those receiving ASC are often vulnerable and like the familiarity of the same carers (i.e., individuals) providing a service over time, which is something that builds inter-personal trust. However, care providers themselves were not immune from the virus. Associated illness, death and self-isolation amongst service providers had a major, disrupting influence, undermining interpersonal trust between service provider and client. The current findings also show that this had systemic causes owing to the marketised, tendering processes for ASC delivery in each of the four territorial welfare systems. As noted, these reward the lowest-cost tenders. In turn, this disincentivises care organisations from investing in staff training and career progression and encourages them to pay the minimum legal wage. In consequence, across polities, there is a major staff retention problem.

In liberal welfare states, the nature and extent of universal welfare provision may shape generalised trust with divides between welfare recipients and those who pay for them (Larsen 2007; Jensen and Svendsen 2011). The current study supports this and shows how, during the pandemic, citizen trust varied between different ASC providers in the different mixed economy models of care delivery. Notably, in England, the public trusted charities and voluntary sector providers to deliver social care more (60 per cent) than other organisations. Central government's role in ASC was trusted by only 7 per cent of respondents (Charities Aid Foundation 2020). Similarly, in Northern Ireland 71 per cent of respondents reported trusting charities in ASC delivery (12 per cent higher than in Great Britain, and 14 per cent higher than the Republic of Ireland, CCNI 2020). The Charity Commissioner for Northern Ireland said: "While I know many charities are struggling simply to survive in the unexpected world we're currently living in, it's important to remember just how vital the public are to charities—and the role that trust and confidence plays in running a successful charity, even during a pandemic. A charity that does not have the public's trust and confidence may find it struggles to raise funds, attract volunteers, staff and even beneficiaries, or simply cannot fulfil its charitable objectives" (CCNI 2020, p. 2). The qualities that the respondents identified as most likely to increase their trust and confidence included making a positive impact on the lives of beneficiaries, transparency and accountability, and operating ethically and honestly (CCNI 2020, p. 2).

6. Conclusions

Foremost of the current study findings is the policy-actors' view that the marketised, capitalist practices that allocate ASC contracts to the lowest-cost tenders fail to deliver the most effective welfare. As the foregoing reveals, such practices are also responsible for a series of trust pathologies. In this regard, there is another institutional trust issue that should be noted. It stems from the way the marketised, mixed economy systems force local third-sector and community organisations into competing with one another, rather than collaborating and pooling resources, knowledge and expertise. As one interviewee observed: "it creates difficulties in terms of trust, and it's not what we get commissioned for ... we have to be in a non-competitive place with our members. Being a service deliverer puts you immediately in a place of competition and that's not where any ... organisation should be".

At this juncture, it is appropriate to reflect upon this study's limitations and opportunities for future research. One limitation is that this study does not capture the full impact of the COVID-19 on the provision of ASC in the community. Rather, it provides needed analysis of the emergence of the pandemic and its initial impact through to late-2021. At the time of writing (circa November 2021), the pandemic was ongoing in the UK (with 43,000 new cases of people contracting Coronavirus and 217 deaths recorded in the past twenty-four hours). Future research will be needed to assess the longer-term impact of this global health emergency. Furthermore, we have deliberately concentrated on the situated knowledge of policy actors, notably, managers and workers with third-sector organisations. Further work is needed to explore and understand the views and experiences of those receiving social care. Their views will also be of vital importance in building future resilience against new health emergencies that may emerge over the coming years. Lastly, we have deliberately adopted a social constructivist and interpretivist epistemology—operationalized through qualitative research methods that draw on the situated knowledge of policy actors. As noted, the reason for this is to let these individuals "speak" to us at a critical juncture in modern history with direct quotations from their accounts of the pandemic. Future work will usefully complement this with quantitative survey data and panel studies.

Overall, the present study's findings suggest the need for more interventionist measures to boost trust in order to deliver higher-quality adult social care in the face of ever-increasing demand. In this regard, there is some evidence that this message is beginning to be taken seriously by politicians and policymakers. For example, according to the Expert Advisory Panel's Proposals to reboot adult care and support in Northern Ireland (Kelly and Kennedy 2017, p. 64), trust and transparency need to be at the heart of a reformed system: "There is a lack of honesty and transparency created by an arms-length commissioning system which is unsuited for the imperfect market that exists in care and support services. It is not the same as procuring stationery or roads maintenance. Care and support involve supporting a human environment and culture that encourages relationships and kindness. The market we create needs to recognise this". Notably, the Scottish discourse also makes the case for addressing these issues through a formal statement of principles—or 'social covenant'—to shape post-pandemic reform: "One key factor is the need for mutual commitment by citizens, representative bodies, providers, civic Scotland, and national government to set aside self-interest and each work together for the common good. Trust is not currently in plentiful supply in social care support and so we believe that there is a need for an explicit social covenant to which all parties would sign up. This will be particularly important if we want to achieve our aspiration for everyone in Scotland to get the social care support they need to live their lives as they choose and to be active citizens" (Scottish Government 2021, p. 13). Whether such measures are part of future ASC reforms will ultimately be determined not by political rhetoric but by the economic necessities of a historically unprecedented post-pandemic fiscal deficit and whether voters are willing to pay the higher taxes such reforms may entail. Past experience does not bode well in this regard.

Author Contributions: Conceptualization, methodology, validation, formal analysis, investigation, resources, data curation, writing—original draft preparation/writing—review and editing, visualization, supervision, project administration—P.C. and C.S. All authors have read and agreed to the published version of the manuscript.

Funding: This research was funded by the Economic and Social Research Council (ESRC), grant number ES/S012435/1. The APC was funded by Hong Kong Baptist University.

Institutional Review Board Statement: The study was conducted according to the guidelines of the Declaration of Helsinki and approved by the Ethics Committee of the School of Social Sciences, Cardiff University. (Protocol code SREC/3417 and 31 January 2017).

Informed Consent Statement: Informed consent was obtained from all subjects involved in the study.

Data Availability Statement: Data supporting reported results will be deposited with the ESRC data archive https://www.data-archive.ac.uk/ (accessed 5 November 2021).

Acknowledgments: The authors are indebted to the editors and three anonymous referees for their helpful and constructive feedback and suggestions on an earlier draft of this paper.

Conflicts of Interest: The authors declare no conflict of interest.

References

Arts, Wil, and John Gelissen. 2002. Three worlds of welfare capitalism or more? A state-of-the-art report. *Journal of European Social Policy* 12: 137–56. [CrossRef]

Asmorowati, Sulikah, Violeta Schubert, and Ayu Puspita Ningrum. 2021. Policy capacity, local autonomy, and human agency: Tensions in the intergovernmental coordination in Indonesia's social welfare response amid the COVID-19 pandemic. *Journal of Asian Public Policy*, 1–15. [CrossRef]

Atkinson, Carol, Sarah Crozier, and Elizabeth Lewis. 2016. *Factors that Affect the Recruitment and Retention of Domiciliary Care Workers and the Extent to Which These Factors Impact Upon the Quality of Domiciliary Care*. Cardiff: Welsh Government.

Basit, Tehmina. 2003. Manual or electronic? The role of coding in qualitative data analysis. *Educational Research* 45: 143–54. [CrossRef]

Borghi, Vando, and Rik Van Berkel. 2007. New Modes of Governance in Italy and the Netherlands: The Case of Activation Policies. *Public Administration* 85: 83–101. [CrossRef]

Bowen, Glenn A. 2009. Document Analysis as a Qualitative Research Method. *Qualitative Research Journal* 9: 27–40. [CrossRef]

Campbell, Steve, Melanie Greenwood, Sarah Prior, Toniele Shearer, Kerrie Walkem, Sarah Young, Danielle Bywaters, and Kim Walker. 2020. Purposive sampling: Complex or simple? Research case examples. *Journal of research in Nursing* 25: 652–61. [CrossRef]

Care Quality Commission. 2019. *The State of Health Care and Adult Social Care in England 2018/19*. Newcastle: Care Quality Commission.

Chaney, Paul. 2020a. Human Rights and Social Welfare Pathologies: Civil Society Perspectives on Contemporary Practice across UK Jurisdictions. *International Journal of Human Rights* 25: 639–74. [CrossRef]

Chaney, Paul. 2020b. Examining Political Parties' Record on Refugees and Asylum Seekers in UK Party Manifestos 1964-2019: The Rise of Territorial Approaches to Welfare? *Journal of Immigrant & Refugee Studies* 19: 488–510.

Chaney, Paul. 2021. Exploring the Politicisation and Territorialisation of Adult Social Care in the UK: Electoral Discourse Analysis of State-wide and Meso Elections 1998–2019. *Global Social Policy*. [CrossRef]

Charities Aid Foundation. 2020. *Giving Civil Society the Right Response: National Policy Responses for Supporting Philanthropy, Giving and Civil Society across the World in the Context of COVID-19*. London: CAF.

Charity Commission of Northern Ireland. 2020. *NICVA COVID-19 Impact Survey 2020*. Belfast: CCNI.

Coalition of Care and Support Providers in Scotland. 2020. *Independent Review of Adult Social Care, Submission from CCPS—Coalition of Care & Support Providers in Scotland*. Edinburgh: CCPS.

Cunningham, Ian, Alina Baluch, Philip James, Eva Jendro, and Douglas Young. 2019. *Handing Back Contracts: Exploring the Rising Trend in Third Sector Provider Withdrawal from the Social Care Market*. Edinburgh: CCPS/University of Strathclyde Business School.

Daniele, Gianmarco, and Benny Geys. 2015. Interpersonal trust and welfare state support. *European Journal of Political Economy* 39: 1–12. [CrossRef]

Department for Digital, Culture, Media and Sport and Office for Civil Society. 2021. *Investigation into Government Funding to Charities during the COVID-19 Pandemic*. London: DCMS.

Dickinson, Helen, Kerry Allen, Pete Alcock, Rob Macmillan, and Jon Glasby. 2012. *The Role of the Third Sector in Delivering Social Care*. London: National Institute for Health Research.

Druckman, James. 2001. The implications of framing effects for citizen competence. *Political Behavior* 23: 225–56. [CrossRef]

Eden, Colin, and Fran Ackermann. 2004. Cognitive Mapping Expert Views for Policy Analysis in the Public Sector. *European Journal of Operational Research* 152: 615–30. [CrossRef]

Esping-Andersen, Gosta. 1990. *The Three Worlds of Welfare Capitalism*. Princeton: Princeton University Press.

Fereday, Jennifer, and Eimear Muir-Cochrane. 2006. Demonstrating Rigor Using Thematic Analysis: A Hybrid Approach of Inductive and Deductive Coding and Theme Development. *International Journal of Qualitative Methods* 5: 80–92. [CrossRef]

Godwill, Engwa A. 2015. *Fundamentals of Research Methodology: A Holistic Guide for Research Completion, Management, Validation and Ethics*. New York: Nova Publishers.

Goffman, Erving. 1974. *Frame Analysis*. Cambridge: Harvard University Press.

Habibov, Nazim, Alena Auchynnikava, Rong Luo, and Lida Fan. 2019. Influence of interpersonal and institutional trusts on welfare state support revisited: Evidence from 27 post-communist nations. *The International Journal of Sociology and Social Policy* 39: 644–60. [CrossRef]

Heine, Bernd, and Heiko Narrog. 2015. *The Oxford Handbook of Linguistic Analysis*, 2nd ed. Oxford: Oxford University Press.

Henderson, Ailsa, Charlie Jeffery, Daniel Wincott, and Richard Wyn Jones. 2013. Reflections on the "devolution paradox": A comparative examination of multilevel citizenship. *Regional Studies* 47: 303–22. [CrossRef]

ICF. 2018a. *The Economic Value of the Adult Social Care Sector—England: Final Report*. London: ICF.

ICF. 2018b. *The Economic Value of the Adult Social Care Sector—Northern Ireland: Final Report*. London: ICF.

ICF. 2018c. *The Economic Value of the Adult Social Care Sector—Scotland: Final Report*. London: ICF.

IFC Consulting. 2018. *The Economic Value of the Adult Social Care Sector—Wales, Final Report*. London: IFC.

James, Allison. 2013. Seeking the analytic imagination: Reflections on the process of interpreting qualitative data. *Qualitative Research* 13: 562–77. [CrossRef]

Jensen, Carsten, and Gert Tinggaard Svendsen. 2011. Giving money to strangers: European welfare states and social trust. *International Journal of Social Welfare* 20: 3–9. [CrossRef]

Kelly, Des, and John Kennedy. 2017. *Power to the People, Proposals to Reboot Adult Care & Support in Northern Ireland*. Belfast: Expert Advisory Panel on Adult Care and Support.

Kevins, Anthony. 2019. Dualized trust: Risk, social trust and the welfare state. *Socio-Economic Review* 17: 875–97. [CrossRef]

Knack, Stephen, and Philip Keefer. 1997. Does social capital have an economic payoff? A cross-country investigation. *Quarterly Journal of Economics* 112: 1251–88. [CrossRef]

Kukla, André. 2000. *Social Constructivism and the Philosophy of Science*. London: Routledge.

Larsen, Christian. 2007. How Welfare Regimes Generate and Erode Social Capital: The Impact of Underclass Phenomena. *Comparative Politics* 40: 83–101. [CrossRef]

Mackieson, Penny, Aron Shlonsky, and Marie Connolly. 2019. Increasing rigor and reducing bias in qualitative research: A document analysis of parliamentary debates using applied thematic analysis. *Qualitative Social Work* 18: 965–80. [CrossRef]

MacPhail, Catherine, Nomhle Khoza, Laurie Abler, and Meghna Ranganathan. 2015. Process guidelines for establishing Intercoder Reliability in qualitative studies. *Qualitative Research* 16: 198–212. [CrossRef]

Mattimoe, Ruth, Michael T. Hayden, Brid Murphy, and Joan Ballantine. 2021. Approaches to Analysis of Qualitative Research Data: A Reflection on the Manual and Technological Approaches. *Accounting, Finance, & Governance Review* 27: 54–69.

National Audit Office. 2021. *The Adult Social Care Market in England*. London: NAO.
Natow, Rebecca S. 2020. The use of triangulation in qualitative studies employing elite interviews. *Qualitative Research* 20: 160–73. [CrossRef]
Northern Ireland Executive Department for Health. 2020. *Department of Health—Temporary Amendment of the Health and Social Care Framework Document for the Period June 2020 to May 2022: Consultation Document*. Belfast: Northern Ireland Executive Department for Health.
Office for National Statistics. 2020. *Population Estimates for the UK, England and Wales, Scotland and Northern Ireland, Provisional: Mid-2019*. Newport: ONS.
Public Health England. 2020. *Beyond the Data: Understanding the Impact of COVID-19 on BAME Groups*. London: PHE.
Rose, Richard. 1991. Is American public policy exceptional? In *Is America Different? A New Look at American Exceptionalism*. Edited by Bercovitch E. Shafer. Oxford: Clarendon Press.
Rothstein, Bo. 1998. *Just Institutions Matter: The Moral and Political Logic of the Universal Welfare State*. Cambridge: Cambridge University Press.
Salamon, Lester M., and Helmut K. Anheier. 1998. Social Origins of Civil Society: Explaining the Nonprofit Sector Cross-Nationally. *VOLUNTAS: International Journal of Voluntary and Nonprofit Organizations* 9: 213–48. [CrossRef]
Saldaña, Johnny. 2021. *The Coding Manual for Qualitative Researchers*, 4th ed. Los Angeles and London: SAGE Publications Ltd.
Scottish Council for Voluntary Organization (SCVO). 2020a. *Manifesto for the Future: A Summary of the SCVO Policy Forum's Blueprint for Scotland*. Edinburgh: SCVO.
Scottish Council for Voluntary Organization (SCVO). 2020b. *Submission to the House of Lords: Lessons from Coronavirus*. Edinburgh: SCVO.
Scottish Government. 2019. *Social Care Support: An Investment in Scotland's People, Society, and Economy—Programme Framework, A Partnership Programme to Support Local Reform of Adult Social Care*. Edinburgh: Scottish Government.
Scottish Government. 2021. *Independent Review of Adult Social Care in Scotland*; Edinburgh: Scottish Government.
Scottish Parliament Equality and Human Rights Committee. 2021. *Report on the Impact of the COVID-19 Pandemic on Equalities and Human Rights*. Edinburgh: Scottish Parliament.
Scottish Parliament. 2013. *Self-Directed Support (Scotland) Act (2013)*. Edinburgh: Scottish Parliament.
Stoetzler, Marcel, and Nira Yuval-Davis. 2002. Standpoint Theory, Situated Knowledge and the Situated Imagination. *Feminist Theory* 3: 315–33. [CrossRef]
Stratton, Samuel J. 2021. Population Research: Convenience Sampling Strategies. *Prehospital and disaster Medicine* 36: 373–74. [CrossRef]
Taylor-Gooby, Peter, ed. 2000. *Risk, Trust and Welfare*. Basingstoke: Palgrave Macmillan.
Uslaner, Eric M. 2002. *The Moral Foundations of Trust*. Cambridge: Cambridge University Press.
Van de Walle, Steven, and Lihi Lahat. 2017. Do Public Officials Trust Citizens? A Welfare State Perspective. *Social Policy & Administration* 51: 1450–69.
Welsh Parliament. 2021. *Equality, Local Government and Communities Committee: Review of the Impact of Covid-19 on the Voluntary Sector*. Cardiff: Welsh Parliament.
Welsh Parliament/Senedd Cymru. 2021. *Health, Social Care and Sport Committee Inquiry into the Impact of the Covid-19 Outbreak, and Its Management, on Health and Social care in Wales*. Cardiff: Welsh Parliament/Senedd Cymru.
Wigell, Mikael. 2017. Political Effects of Welfare Pluralism: Comparative Evidence from Argentina and Chile. *World Development* 95: 27–42. [CrossRef]
Wimmer, Andreas, and Nina Glick Schiller. 2002. Methodological nationalism and beyond: Nation–State building, migration and the social sciences. *Global Networks* 2: 301–34. [CrossRef]
Wong, Timothy Ka-ying, Po-san Wan, and Hsin-Huang Michael Hsiao. 2011. The bases of political trust in six Asian societies: Institutional and cultural explanations compared. *International Political Science Review* 32: 263–81. [CrossRef]

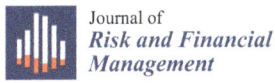

Journal of
Risk and Financial Management

Communication

Trust, Transparency and Transnational Lessons from COVID-19

Alistair Cole [1], Julien S. Baker [2] and Dionysios Stivas [1,*]

1 Department of Government and International Studies, Hong Kong Baptist University, Kowloon Tong 999077, Hong Kong; alistaircole@hkbu.edu.hk
2 Centre for Health and Exercise Science Research, Department of Sport, Physical Education and Health, Hong Kong Baptist University, Kowloon Tong 999077, Hong Kong; jsbaker@hkbu.edu.hk
* Correspondence: stivasd@hkbu.edu.hk

Abstract: The article engages in an exercise in reflexivity around trust and the COVID-19 pandemic. Common understandings of trust are mapped out across disciplinary boundaries and discussed in the cognitive fields in the medical and social sciences. While contexts matter in terms of the understandings and uses made of concepts such as trust and transparency, comparison across academic disciplines and experiences drawn from country experiences allows general propositions to be formulated for further exploration. International health crises require efforts to rebuild trust, understood in a multidisciplinary sense as a relationship based on trusteeship, in the sense of mutual obligations in a global commons, where trust is a key public good. The most effective responses in a pandemic are joined up ones, where individuals (responsible for following guidelines) trust intermediaries (health professionals) and are receptive to messages (nudges) from the relevant governmental authorities. Hence, the distinction between hard medical and soft social science blurs when patients and citizens are required to be active participants in combatting the virus. Building on the diagnosis of a crisis of trust (in the field of health security and across multiple layers of governance), the article renews with calls to restore trust by enhancing transparency.

Keywords: COVID-19; coronavirus disease; trust; transparency; political trust; social trust; transnational; transdisciplinary

Citation: Cole, Alistair, Julien S. Baker, and Dionysios Stivas. 2021. Trust, Transparency and Transnational Lessons from COVID-19. *Journal of Risk and Financial Management* 14: 607. https://doi.org/10.3390/jrfm14120607

Academic Editor: Thanasis Stengos

Received: 28 November 2021
Accepted: 13 December 2021
Published: 15 December 2021

Publisher's Note: MDPI stays neutral with regard to jurisdictional claims in published maps and institutional affiliations.

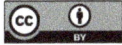

Copyright: © 2021 by the authors. Licensee MDPI, Basel, Switzerland. This article is an open access article distributed under the terms and conditions of the Creative Commons Attribution (CC BY) license (https://creativecommons.org/licenses/by/4.0/).

1. Introduction

Responding to existential dilemmas, the COVID-19 pandemic calls for a major transdisciplinary research effort that necessarily combines several levels of empirical analysis and methodological tools (statistical, experimental, qualitative, comparative, interpretative) and bridges distinct academic and scientific traditions. The questions raised by COVID-19 are germane to the medical and the social sciences. From an international relations perspective, COVID-19 gets to the heart of what comprises a common good—the global commons. From a public policy perspective, COVID-19 is the wicked policy problem par excellence, requiring interagency collaboration. From a comparative politics perspective, COVID-19 provides a vast living dataset to engage in multilevel comparisons and real-time experiments. In the medical research field, the pandemic has provided advancements in medical science that would not have been possible without access to a living laboratory. However, the advancement in knowledge related to the pandemic may have been further accelerated if the local and international communities and policy makers were united in their administrative approach. By linking the medical and social sciences, through the distinct prism of trust, the article contributes to reflections upon the COVID-19 pandemic.

The article engages in a transnational and transdisciplinary exercise in reflexivity around the theme of trust and COVID-19. This scoping article is centered on the question of whether the COVID-19 pandemic represents, inter alia, a crisis of trust, one theme that successfully travels between the social and medical sciences. The article does not attempt to process trace public policy in relation to COVID-19 as a result of public policy. Any attempt to do so, would be extremely complicated to achieve. Process-tracing involving study-based empirical analysis might allow inferences in relation to a specific country case; but could not easily be replicated. Mapping statistical indicators in a comparative sense lies beyond the scope of this article. As (Cole and Stivas 2020) have demonstrated (Table 1), trust is deeply contextual. Interpretation is the best way forward, in the context where outcomes cannot be known. Outputs, on the other hand, can be interpreted. Meijer et al. (2018), for example, provide an interpretative framework to guide and structure assessments of government transparency. Moreover, the imposing body of literature that has been published on trust and transparency is targeted at processes and possibly outputs. Lægreid and Rykkja (2019) connect successful crisis management with the citizens' behavior that is based on trust in government and on government capacity. Boin et al. (2017) suggest that to assess the crisis response, one must, among others, ask how prepared the authorities were, and how they made sense of the crisis and communicated with citizens. The article maps out common understandings of trust across disciplinary boundaries and discusses how these might be applied to cognitive fields in the medical and social sciences.

Table 1. Trust, transparency and control of COVID-19 in China, the U.K., Taiwan, and Hong Kong (as of 31 January 2021).

	Mode of Governance	Political Trust	Trust in Experts	Transparency	Deaths and Cases/1 Million Population
China (Mainland)	Authoritarian	High	High	Low	Deaths/1 million: 3 Cases/1 million: 62
U.K.	Democratic	Medium	High	Medium	Deaths/1 million: 1550 Cases/1 million: 55,748
Taiwan	Democratic	High	High	High	Deaths/1 million: 0.3 Cases/1 million: 38
Hong Kong SAR	Hybrid Democracy	Low	High	High	Deaths/1 million: 24 Cases/1 million: 1381

Building on the diagnosis of a crisis of trust in the field of health security and governance (Downs and Larson 2007; Hilyard et al. 2010; Lo Yuk-ping and Thomas 2010), the article renews with calls to restore trust (thereby improving understandings of the challenges raised by COVID-19) by enhancing transparency. Section One introduces a brief review of the core dimensions of trust and COVID-19, while section two develops a multi-layered, transnational and transdisciplinary inquiry. In the final section, the authors provide pointers for how to rebuild trust by restoring an optimum trust balance.

2. A Question of Trust

Trust has long been identified as an essential component of social, economic and political life (Cook 2001; Rothstein 2005). Earle and Siegrist identify trust as the willingness to make oneself vulnerable to another based on a judgement of similarity of intentions or values (2008). The wider trust literature has identified a range of potential factors underpinning trust, such as citizen satisfaction with policy, economic performance, the prevalence of political scandals and corruption and the influence of social capital. Parker et al. (2014, p. 87) sum up the underlying assumption in much of the literature that 'the public is more trusting when they are satisfied with policy outcomes, the economy is booming, citizens are pleased with incumbents and institutions, political scandals are nonexistent, crime is low, a war is popular, the country is threatened, and social capital is high.' There is also a frequent link with mistrust, though the latter phenomenon also has its own distinct literature (Avery 2009; Davis 1976; Fraser 1970; Sztompka 2006). Health scandals, such as mad cow disease in the UK or the tainted blood scandal in France, have a particular place in the interface between citizens and their trust in politics and the health and related professions (Lanska 1998). In the current literature, trust is treated as one of the main determinants of citizens' compliance and collaboration with the governmental measures during a pandemic (Balog-Way and McComas 2020; Rowe and Calnan 2006;

Slovic 1999). Considering trust and the COVID-19 pandemic, Fetzer et al. (2020) associated the high levels of trust in government with the low levels of stress and misperceptions. They concluded that high levels of trust generated higher degrees of compliance with the governmental measures. Similar were the findings of Oksanen et al. (2020) who studied the relationship between trust and compliance in various countries of Europe.

There are powerful causal narratives around the loss of trust in contemporary societies. Four types of explanation are typically provided for the loss of trust (Devine et al. 2020; IPSOS 2020; Martin et al. 2020; Seyd 2020). Is the loss of trust a consequence of poor performance (after a decade of sluggish economic growth and inability to recover from the financial crisis of 2008–09) (van der Meer and Hakhverdian 2017)? Or is it the result of a disconnect and distance between government and citizens, with the former unable to accommodate the preferences of the latter (Fledderus et al. 2014; Fisher et al. 2010; Hardin 2002)? Or does it result from a general belief that politicians in general are corrupt and self-serving (Grimmelikhuijsen 2012; Park and Blenkinsopp 2011)? Or, indeed, is it the consequence of a lack of transparency and accountability? These four dimensions—trust and performance, trust and disconnect, trust and honesty or benevolence, trust and transparency—are each pertinent as forms of bridging research agendas. These precise linkages are explored here in terms of the health and security crisis represented by COVID-19.

Trust and performance: Is trust a consequence of 'output legitimacy' whereby users reward or punish service providers on account of results? In many countries, there has been a diffusion of new public management-type solutions in health care, whereby services are evaluated on the basis of key performance indicators such as the number of operations delivered or beds occupied. A holistic view of healthcare has, arguably, suffered (Kruk and Freedman 2008; Veillard et al. 2005). Financial resources (30–35% of budgets) invested in medical care have been diverted into human resources involved in a myriad of administrative tasks (Shrank et al. 2019). The narrative of performance runs counter to the absolute belief in healthcare. Part of the problem is one of process: how effectively are resources devoted to frontline services? Hence, in France there is controversy over organizations such as the regional health agencies, run by technocrats rather than professionals, on the basis of 'managerial' performance indicator regimes. While this can be interpreted in terms of corporate defense on behalf of the medical profession, it is also the case that narrow key performance indicators do not lend themselves to more holistic risk management strategies. There were controversies in several countries, at the height of the pandemic, over the lack of medical supplies because of outsourcing and the negative consequences of management by objectives (allegedly reducing the number of beds available for COVID-19 emergency patients). Such disputes did little to reduce mistrust between governments and citizens.

Trust and disconnect: The pandemic has revealed how administrative complexity can be an independent factor of mistrust. Who does what is a vital question in terms of basic transparency. Competition between bureaus can have a debilitating effect in terms of access to public services, especially during a period of pandemic. In the case of France, for example, how to obtain masks, gloves, sprays, or simply to undertake a test involved intense interagency (regional health agency, prefectures) and intergovernmental (the state against the regions) competition. Similar stories emerged elsewhere, not least between the central government and the devolved administrations in the UK or the central government and the autonomous communities in Spain. This issue is not a simple one of distinction between types of polity, for example federal versus unitary systems: while the US and Brazilian federations descended into partisan-based rivalries between states, federal Germany initially demonstrated one of the most joined-up responses to the pandemic.

Trust and honesty or benevolence: Health professionals have been in the forefront of the fight against COVID-19, but they are not always free to tell the truth. Scientific communities themselves are divided, adding to the contested status of scientific truth. From the perspective of medical practitioners, questions of distributive justice (Huxtable 2020)—about the allocation of resources and the determination of which patients should receive treatment—are paramount, yet difficult to assume politically, hence the link to questions of transparency.

Trust and transparency: The presupposition that transparency produces better outcomes underpins much contemporary policy. Transparency might also be framed in terms of building confidence via accountability and participation and enhancing trust on account of fairness and open procedures. Heald (2013) outlines four directions of transparency: vertical transparency (where a person or an organization has hierarchical oversight over another person or organization), upwards transparency (when the superior can observe the subordinate), downwards transparency (where the rulers are accountable to the ruled), and horizontal transparency (further elaborated by Grimmelikhuijsen 2012, p. 563) as 'the availability of information about an organization'). Unpicking Heald's model, and applying its approach to COVID-19, there are variable linkages to trust and transparency across time and space. Vertical transparency and upwards transparency can be combined. They appear as a modern equivalent of Bentham's panopticon, where the central guardians (of a prison, of the state) can observe and thereby control all activities of subordinates. Such data-intensive and intrusive mechanisms have come to the fore during the COVID-19 crisis, as governments have resorted to extraordinary measures to 'securitize' the pandemic. Such measures are possibly efficient and probably necessary, especially when physical movement needs to be limited. Such methods have not been limited to authoritarian regimes, but they have spilled over into more general use in Western democracies (worn down by the past decade of terrorist attacks). Blurred processes, emergency procedures and a constitutional decision-making circuit have scarcely ensured clear information about how crisis decisions were reached during the pandemic. They have fallen down against the standard of trust as honesty and diminished the bases of freedom. They are unlikely to build trust. In Hong Kong, for instance, despite the local government's attempts to persuade the public that its dealings with the pandemic are transparent (the government explicitly emphasized transparency in official statements, activated COVID-19-relevant information proxies, and conducted daily press conferences), the trust in Hong Kong government is amongst the lowest globally. How the different 'directions' of transparency intervene with the 'levels' and 'determinants' of trust is illustrated in Figure 1. We assume that transparency can influence trust mostly at the 'trust in government' level of trust and therefore, in a downwards direction of transparency. To support our arguments, we build on the most up-to-date literature on COVID-19. We substantiate our claims with evidence from various administrations and we highlight notable events from each administration's struggle to control the pandemic.

Throughout the article, we make the point that trust as performance, connection, benevolence and transparency is most effective when these facets are combined. Specifically, we do not rank these values or prioritize transparency. We focus more on transparency, however, in part because of content and word limitations, in part because of the growing couplings of the two concepts (Cucciniello et al. 2017) but mainly because it is the best one for distinguishing between national responses.

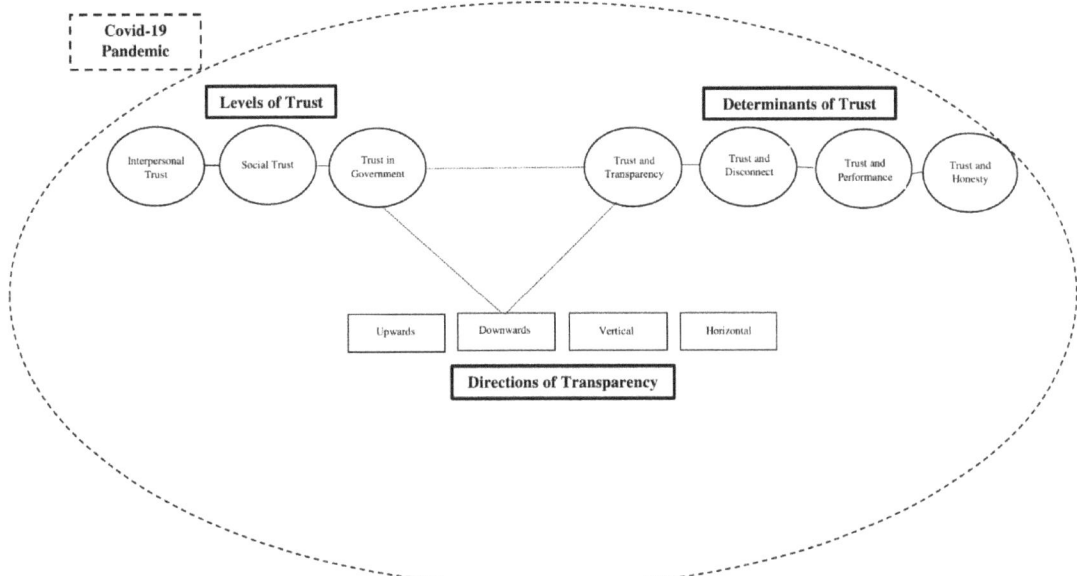

Figure 1. Directions of transparency, levels and determinants of trust.

3. Trust, COVID-19 and Transdisciplinary Enquiry

The social scientist is bound to defer in some respects to the medical sciences, but each has an interest in conceptualizing the role of trust and mistrust during health crises. The agendas are genuinely transdisciplinary. There has been mass mobilization: from governments, research agencies, big pharmaceutical firms, professional bodies, the medical, scientific and artificial intelligence communities, all in search of problem solutions and understanding. No interest has been left unaffected, be it in international organizations (the World Health Organization, the European Union), powerful nations (United States, China), multinational firms, the professions, civil society and individuals.

The pandemic demonstrates the contested nature of medical knowledge: as testified by the early controversies over hydroxychloroquine, through the race for a vaccine, or contrasting containment strategies (herd immunity against lockdown and, more recently, zero-cases against endemic virus approaches). Scientists have replaced politicians as regular guests of radio and 24 h television programs. However, the crisis also illustrates the barriers to the functioning of a global medical epistemic community, free to exchange in the interests of scientific discovery.

The article interrogates one dimension of the health crisis: namely, the role of trust. Trust is one of the most contested concepts within academic research. The OECD (2017, p. 3) has argued that 'governments cannot function effectively without the trust of citizens, nor can they successfully carry out public policies, notably more ambitious reform agendas.' Elsewhere we have defined trust in terms of human-like constructs such as relationships (interpersonal, intermediate, institutional), properties (benevolence, honesty, ability, trustworthiness), levels (interpersonal, social, institutional, international), types (confidential, community), in relation to associated concepts (resilience, risk, confidence, transparency), and in terms of public policy and processes (Stafford et al. 2022). For current purposes, trust needs to be understood as a generic term to describe dynamics taking place at different levels of analysis: interpersonal, social and collective. The trust literature allows a fairly precise operationalization, especially relating to the three levels of trust of Zmerli and Newton (2011), which can be adapted to the COVID-19 crisis. Medical and social science rely on theorizing at three main levels of analysis: individual, intermediate and institutional. Each type of analysis carries a distinctive contribution and the stakes of each are high, including psychological wellbeing, a civil society and trust in government.

Interpersonal trust: Rousseau et al. (1998, p. 395) define trust as 'a psychological state comprising the intention to accept vulnerability based upon positive expectations of the intentions or behavior of another'. It involves an interpersonal relationship, with at least two players, as in a clinical–patient relationship. In terms of both trust and confidence, the individual level is key, because individual perceptions of risk are germane to the adoption of preventive measures (Khosravi 2020). Citing studies of various countries, Siegrist and Zingg (2014, p. 25) suggest that 'trust had a positive impact on adopting precautionary behavior during a pandemic'. In another close formulation 'particular social trust' involves those known to us personally, such as family, friends or work colleagues. A breakdown of trust shatters this psychological equilibrium. Cross-national evidence from lockdowns and quarantines illuminates the challenged state of psychological well-being of individuals, especially in terms of their primary networks (friends, family) and practices (as a result of social distancing). Even within these tight personal networks, evidence from scholars working on psychological indicators points to an increase in indicators of social tension, such as divorce, gender violence and isolation as a result of the COVID-19 crisis (Boserup et al. 2020). Increases in social violence and violation by communities in relation to social distancing measures are major concerns in relation to public perceptions and information provided by respective governments and their representatives. Misinformation and lack of action in the early stages by governments led to an apathetical approach by communities and a feeling of identity immunity that proved costly as the pandemic wore on.

Such tensions are also apparent in the medical/clinical domain. Adapted to medical ethics, for example, practitioner and client relationships span elements of interpersonal and intermediate trust. The appropriate relationship is prescribed and described in medical ethics (with trust as a form of confidential relationship, absolutely secretive, in no senses negotiated with a third party) and regulated by strict professional and ethical standards. Here, the medical relationship is stronger than even the tightest form of inter-personal political relationship. COVID-19 challenges interpersonal (medical) trust in a novel manner; traditional consultative practices are changing (with the rise of eMedecine), while the competition for scarce resources has ensured that COVID-19 has eclipsed more traditional treatments (for example, the postponing of cancer operations).

Recent literature in the field of pediatrics has also raised issues of trust between medical practitioners, children and parents and raised the question of the appropriate level of analysis. At the individual level of analysis, trust is essential to the clinical–family relationship. Trust constitutes more than an intentional action; it involves a confidential relationship. Trusting relationships can produce 'confidence, peace of mind and security, while broken trust breeds stress, game playing and anxiety' (Sisk and Baker 2019, p. 1). The central paradox, in the relationship between pediatricians and children, is that trusting relationships are mediated by third parties, by parents. There is an enormous leap from the individual-level, through socially mediated forms of trust and onto the headline events such as a crisis of trust in the US health system. Sisk and Baker (2019) identify a deeply embedded crisis in doctors and the US health care system as a whole over the last half century, a finding that could be exported to many other countries.

The key analytical point is that, in the medical sphere as in the political one, discussion centers on the linkages between individual, intermediary and organizational levels of analysis. The COVID-19 pandemic has focused attention on the need to strengthen the links between patients, health care teams and organizations. From the relevant literature, we learn that the most effective responses in a pandemic are joined up ones, where individuals (responsible for following guidelines) trust intermediaries (health professionals) and are receptive to messages (nudges) from the relevant governmental authorities. Hence, the distinction between hard medical and soft social science blurs when patients/citizens are required to be active participants in combatting the virus. The two worlds are linked by the questions of trust.

Social or collective trust: 'General social trust' is that placed in 'unknown others'. This form of trust performs a key function in modern societies, as Newton (2007, p. 349) notes, because 'much social interaction is between people who neither know one another nor share a common social background.' Generalized social trust or 'thin trust' is centered on more general information about social groups and situations (Keele 2007). In relation to COVID-19, the ability to empathize with members of an imagined community (region, nation, even continent) is a core element of community integration. Health professionals—frontline workers, such as nurses—are everywhere a source of national pride and mobilization, yet they are also amongst the individuals the most in danger of contracting the virus. How civil society has reacted to the pandemic is a matter of empirical investigation. Social capital is literally excluded, as a result of lockdown and travel restrictions. Society has not collapsed. Even where confinement was harsh, as in Italy, Spain and France, the strength of civil ties allowed the crisis to be weathered. Public participation is central to the success of adopting preventive measures.

There has been a dangerous ebbing of social trust in many countries where the utility of wearing masks was questioned and, above all, where vaccination has been actively contested and resisted. Hence a society's response to the pandemic depends on the levels of trust—trust in civil society, trust in health professionals and trust in the government—and the interactions between these variables. The case of Hong Kong is interesting in this respect. Though the Hong Kong SAR Government was very transparent in providing data about its handling of the virus, it enjoyed relatively low levels of public trust. Nonetheless, the city is widely considered as having been effective in containing the virus. The numbers of COVID-19 infections and deaths are amongst the lowest in the world while, for the duration of the pandemic, Hong Kong never resorted to imposing any severe intracommunity restrictive measures. Hong Kong's successful approach can be traced to the high level of trust in civil society and interpersonal trust among its citizens. Here, there is a slightly paradoxical situation where the trust in the government is not very high, but people are behaving in a way that is cooperative towards the government's measures to curb the spread of the virus (Chan 2021). Hong Kong society showed itself to be disciplined and coherent, as Hong Kongers swiftly adopted mask-wearing in public to illustrate their collective reaction to COVID-19. Mask-wearing was among the risk management measures proposed by the government of Hong Kong. Stronger trust in the risk management authority can facilitate cooperation (Chan 2021; Groeniger et al. 2021; Rieger and Wang 2021). In Hong Kong, despite the low levels of trust to the government, the citizens complied with the mask-wearing rules. This capacity of the community has kept Hong Kong largely unaffected by the pandemic. It is also noteworthy that a high level of trust in health professionals is recorded in Hong Kong (Smith 2020), making it a key determinant of how well Hong Kong contains COVID-19. The general public's response contributed to Hong Kong's low number of COVID-19 cases and deaths.

Trust in government: our third dimension, has performed a major role during the pandemic by affecting the public's judgements about risks and related benefits (Khosravi 2020). From a psychological perspective, Bish and Michie (2010) argue that trust in government is a key variable affecting individual behavior faced with pandemics; the more consistent the message, the more likely it is to influence behavior. Zmerli and Newton (2011, p. 3) define political trust as a 'very thin form of trust' characterized by a 'kind of general expectation that on the whole, political leaders will act according to the rules of the game'. The arguments about the role of trust in the current literature are divided. Some researchers argue that at the beginning of the pandemic and in certain jurisdictions, trust in government was increased (Bol et al. 2021; Groeniger et al. 2021; Rieger and Wang 2021; Sibley et al. 2020). Conversely, indexes of political trust (e.g., the Edelman Trust Barometer (Edelman 2021)) suggest a general decline across liberal democracies in the past decade, even before the COVID-19 crisis. The evidence points to variable dosages of mistrust in different democratic countries, with a typical trust cycle (rallying to the executive, followed by deep unpopularity) being observed as during other pandemics (van der Weerd et al. 2011). Of more importance is the challenge to fundamental liberal-democratic values occasioned by the pandemic. Political anthropologists identify as 'tricksters' characters intent on subverting the system that brought them to power (Horvath et al. 2020). More than one leader has attempted to make 'good use of a crisis', to drive through contested political changes (the case of Hungary's premier Victor Orban being the obvious one). Even when the transgression of democracy has been less explicit, there are fears of a hollowing out of civil society and a weakening of civil liberties, via tracing applications such as *Tous anti-covid* in France or *LeaveHomeSafe* in Hong Kong.

4. Rebuilding Trust by Restoring an Optimum Trust Balance

Often trust is mistakenly presented as confidence and confidence as trust. In their 'Trust, Confidence and Cooperation' model, Earle and Siegrist (2008) distinguish between trust and confidence. Trust is defined as the willingness to make oneself vulnerable to another based on a judgement of similarity of intentions or values. Confidence is defined as the belief based on past experience or evidence that certain events will occur as expected. Both trust and confidence influence people's willingness to cooperate. Binding trust and confidence imply the need for consistent messages from central government, along with authoritative steering from intermediaries such as the health and medical professions. The prospects for such convergence are improved where, as in Hong Kong, there was recent experience of a pandemic and behavior adapted accordingly. Zhu (2020), for example, stressed the importance of the experience that the population of Hong Kong gained with fighting SARS in 2003.

Trust in government is important; even more central is trust and confidence in advisors/experts (Lavazza and Farina 2020). During pandemics, most people are not in a position to evaluate the information about the risks and benefits associated with vaccination. Therefore, they rely on experts, especially on those experts they trust, who are once removed from government. This finding was backed by van der Weerd et al. (2011) in their study of the H1N1 flu pandemic in the Netherlands: most of the respondents wanted the information about infection prevention to come from the municipal health services, health care providers and the media, rather than central government. In some cases (i.e., Hong Kong SAR and Taiwan) experts are mobilized to strengthen the trust in institutions. In other instances, the medical experts are sidelined, or even silenced, by the governmental officials (see the case of the whistle-blowing doctor, Li Wenliang, at the onset of the pandemic in China). It is also possible that the trust between politicians and experts breaks down as it happened with the UK Sage committee, or with the central scientific committee in France. When such conflicts occur, political will prevails. In sum, governments of all persuasions seek the maximum utility from medical experts. However, there can be a tipping point in the relationship between politicians and experts, especially when the experts appear to contradict the government (e.g., the conflict between former US president Trump and Anthony Fauci).

In terms of trust, individual responses and reactions, social mediation and governmental responses need to complement each other. Trust processes are different at each of these levels, but the literature points to their mutually reinforcing character (Anderson 1998; Diez Medrano 1995). In a pandemic, governments need to persuade individuals to adapt their behaviors, and such persuasion will be all the more convincing in that it is nested in social networks. Here, reverting to the advice of psychologists and medical scientists assumes its own coherence. Bringing into coherence the three levels of analysis is the best means for ensuring the diffusion of legible, clear messages, with the potential to build trust based on confidence (Siegrist and Zingg 2014).

The adjectival qualities of trust—performance, connection, benevolence, transparency—are also most effective when combined. Performance is best understood in discursive terms as performativity; coherent speech acts underpinned by consistent reasoning are the best shaped to be able to persuade and make citizens susceptible to nudge. The messages coming from the top need to be consistent within their own terms of reference; far from the governmental cacophony observed in France or the US, or—even worse—the transgressive behavior of advisors in UK. Double standards have a detrimental effect on honesty, hence affect perceptions of benevolence, feed disconnection and political distancing from the people. Blurred and contradictory messages by political leaders and their entourages during the COVID-19 crisis ran counter to the advice of medical practitioners, whereby transparency in terms of access to decisions and to information is the best way of influencing behavior during a pandemic and restoring trust (van der Weerd et al. 2011). Similar conclusions might be deduced from the work view of the transparency optimists working in the field of political science. Grimmelikhuijsen (2012) has shown in an experiment that, while citizens will use performance information to make rational and conscious decisions, the positive effect of transparency on trust is also partly due to an emotional factor related to the act of transparency as such. That government appears to be transparent is in itself a factor of the perceived competence component of trust. Hence, governments need to provide accessible information, while avoiding information overload (van de Walle and Roberts 2008). Clear consistent ethical guidelines are called for by the medical community (Huxtable 2020).

Clear and consistent legitimizing discourses are, almost by definition, most difficult to sustain in a crisis, the political equivalent of Schumpeter's creative destruction. For governments to be consistent in their discourses and actions during a pandemic is not an easy task. In times of crisis, governments assume certain risks. Sometimes they risk to undertake measures that can cause thousands of COVID-19 related deaths in order to spare their administration's economy. Conversely, sometimes, the authorities risk devastating the economic life of their countries by imposing severe and lengthy lockdowns in order to safeguard as many lives as possible (Bol et al. 2021). In other instances, policymakers assume the risk of serving the interests of particular interest groups at the expense of others. Risk assumption is inherent in crises. Risk assumption affects the capability of policymakers to be consistent not only in their rhetoric, but also in their actions.

How can trust in public policy making be established or restored? Many recent examples show how easy it is to lose in public policy making, as the cases of financial policy, pension policy, environmental policy and many other examples demonstrate. Already on shallow foundations, the COVID-19 crisis demonstrated stark national variations between countries. Which factors be identified that support the production of trust? Transparency, as a major phenomenon in its own right (Cucciniello et al. 2017), emerges from recent literature as one of the key factors for the production of trust (Stafford 2017). Regular calls for transparency heard during scandals, where trust is lost, aim at restoring trust and are a case in point. While trust is essential for controlling the virus in an immediate sense, transparency and openness of information is necessary for a longer-term policy response that is resilient and sustainable. The research suggested that maintaining transparency of administrative data is the best way to influence behavior during a pandemic and restore trust. The messages coming from the top need to be clear and consistent. Is transparency thus the principal mechanism for restoring trust? It is not that straightforward. In fact, the case of COVID-19 illustrates a trust-transparency paradox, whereby trust requires transparency (witness the reaction to early attempts to deny the virus and control information), but transparency can undermine trust (insofar as it focuses attention on the malfunctioning of liberal democracies and their uneven management of the crisis). In Figure 2, we build on the trust-transparency matrix of Stafford et al. (2022) to demonstrate the complex relationship between trust and transparency. In China mainland, the surveys reveal that almost the total of the citizenry trust their government (Edelman 2021). At the same time, the openness of the government is limited, if non-existent. We call *Blind Faith* this mix of high trust with low transparency that we observe in China. The Taiwanese government also enjoyed high levels of political trust during the pandemic. However, the authorities of the Pacific island were much more transparent than the authorities in mainland China about their dealings with the pandemic. High trust and high transparency, like in Taiwan, resulted in a *Synergy* between the authorities and the public. Conversely, a combination of low trust and high transparency, as observed in Hong Kong, could result in negligible effects during a pandemic. As aforementioned, although the citizens of Hong Kong distrust their arguably transparent government, the coastal city has effectively controlled COVID-19. We name this situation: *Negligible Effects*. Lastly, a situation of low trust and medium to low transparency, as in the U.K., generates a *Dual Dysfunctionality*.[1] The above cases indicate that neither trust nor transparency are absolute preconditions of effective policymaking. There are more general paradoxes of transparency and trust: healthcare workers are the most trusted, for example, and the media least. Yet, in the era of 24-hour media coverage, strengthened by confinement, the media is the main source of information and performs a key transparency role in liberal democracies.

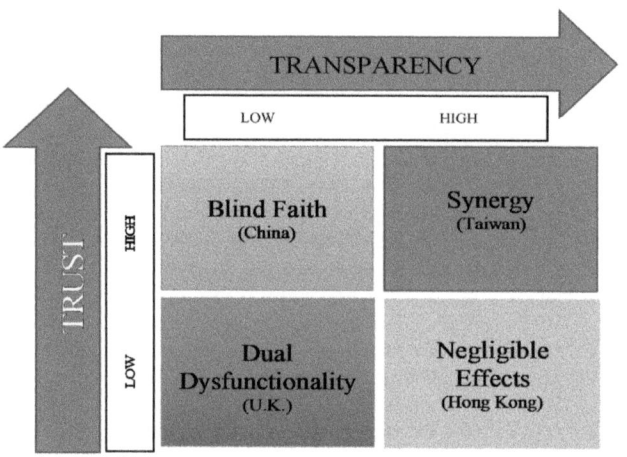

Figure 2. Trust-transparency matrix.

Unlike trust, the dimensions of transparency do not all push in the same direction. Vertical and upwards transparency are particularly suited to authoritarian regimes, or to executive-led decision-making processes (relying on emergency procedures and unaccountable uses of technology) in democratic regimes. Such regimes, turned inwards, are unlikely to embrace transparency beyond a form of social and political control: hence, the unwillingness to consent to the requirement to combat a global pandemic, to engage in policy transfer, to trust a global commons or to accept international standards, akin to international accounting norms. This lack of transparency feeds international mistrust: the pandemic demonstrated widespread skepticism of the validity of statistics across nations, for example. The trust-transparency linkage makes most sense in the context of downwards and horizontal transparency. Restoring global norm-based governance requires commitment to the most positive elements of the transparency agenda, in terms of agreed international standards (for example, over health statistics), engagement with existing international organizations (especially the World Health Organization) and drawing the most robust knowledge from transdisciplinary scientific approaches. Global norms are more important than ever. International health crises require efforts to rebuild trust, understood in a multidisciplinary sense as a relationship based on trusteeship, in the sense of mutual obligations in a global commons, where trust is a key public good.

Author Contributions: A.C. mainly wrote the manuscript; J.S.B. and D.S. mainly contributed to discussion and editing. All authors have read and agreed to the published version of the manuscript.

Funding: This research was funded by the Hung Hin Shiu Charitable Foundation 孔憲紹慈善基金贊助 by the Hong Kong Baptist University Research Committee (Project 165234), by the Hong Kong

Baptist University, Research Committee, Initiation Grant—Faculty Niche Research Areas (IG-FNRA) 2019/20 and by the Heinrich Boell Stiftung.

Data Availability Statement: Not applicable.

Acknowledgments: We acknowledge all the presenters and participants of the conference "Transnational and transdisciplinary lessons of COVID-19 from the perspective of risk and management". We thank Ian Stafford of Cardiff University for advising on the trust-transparency matrix in Figure 2 and generally providing an expert overview.

Conflicts of Interest: The authors declare no conflict of interest.

Appendix A

Measuring Trust and Trasnparency in China, Taiwan, Hong Kong, and the UK

To measure political trust, we consulted large-N surveys conducted by Edelman, YouGov and PORI. The data gathered by these public opinion polls is consistent (they collect their data in various specified jurisdictions and at regular time intervals) and reliable. We adapt Edelman's classification of trust to classify trust higher than 60% as 'trust', between 50% and 59% as 'neutral', and under 49% as 'distrust'. When it comes to transparency, we also set three levels: transparent, neutral, and nontransparent. Since there is no common definition of transparency and its determinants in the current literature, we set up our own scale and pointers. We treat the presence, methods, and frequency of official communication regarding the cases, fatalities and measures related to the epidemic as indicators of transparency. Who makes the announcements is also essential as governments engage health experts to make public announcements in order to enhance the chances of public cooperation. E-involvement of the public in the decision making about the measures necessary to control the virus is another marker of transparency. We draw information about transparency from official governmental data, sources, communications, and academic literature. The results of our inquiry of trust and transparency in the UK, China, Hong Kong, and Taiwan are visualized in the following graphs.

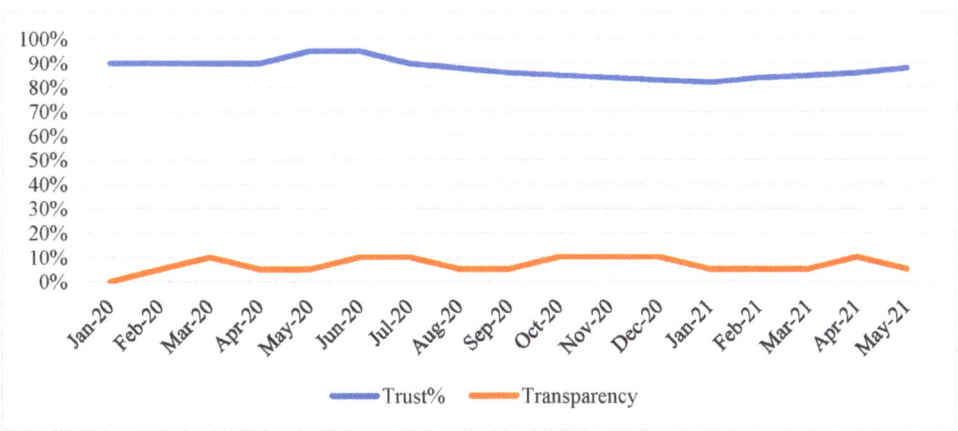

Figure A1. Trust and transparency in mainland China. Source: Edelman Barometer (Edelman 2021) and authors' appraisal of transparency.

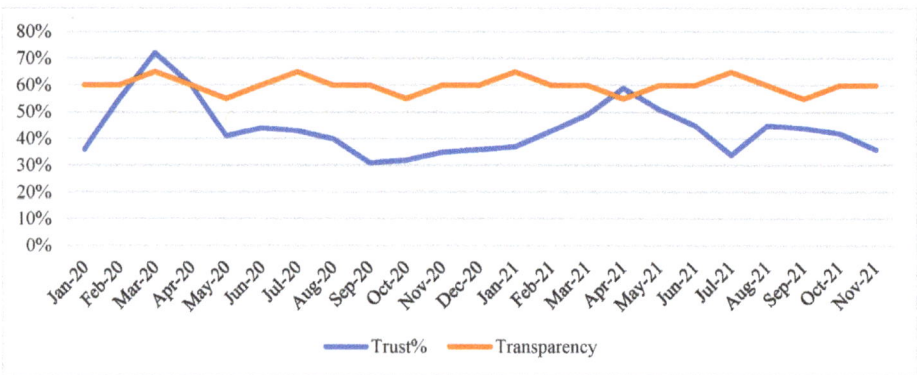

Figure A2. Trust and transparency in the UK. Source: Edelman Barometer (Edelman 2021), YouGov (2021) and authors' appraisal of transparency.

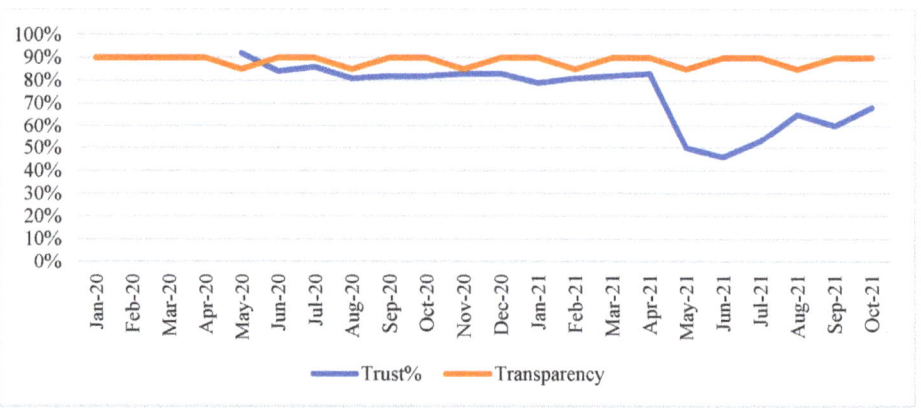

Figure A3. Trust and transparency in Taiwan. Source: YouGov (2021) and authors' appraisal of transparency.

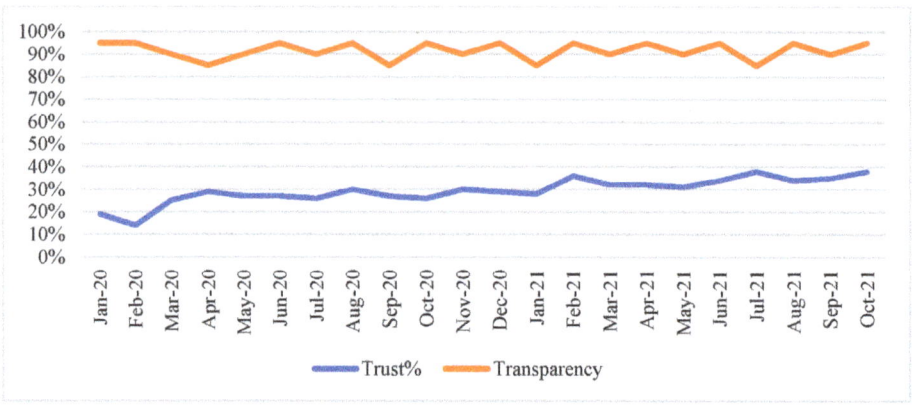

Figure A4. Trust and transparency in Hong Kong. Source: PORI (2021) and authors' appraisal of transparency.

Notes

1 Details, conceptualization, and visualization of trust and transparency in the four administrations, and in the context of the COVID-19 pandemic, are provided in the Appendix A.

References

Anderson, Christopher J. 1998. When in Doubt, Use Proxies: Attitudes toward Domestic Politics and Support for European Integration. *Comparative Political Studies* 31: 569–601. [CrossRef]
Avery, James M. 2009. Political Mistrust among African Americans and Support for the Political System. *Political Research Quarterly* 62: 132–45. [CrossRef]
Balog-Way, Dominic P.H., and Katherine A. McComas. 2020. COVID-19: Reflections on trust, tradeoffs, and preparedness. *Journal of Risk Research* 23: 838–48. [CrossRef]
Bish, Alison, and Susan Michie. 2010. Demographic and attitudinal determinants of protective behaviours during a pandemic: A review. *British Journal of Health Psychology* 15: 797–824. [CrossRef] [PubMed]
Bol, Damien, Marco Giani, Ander Blais, and Peter John Loewen. 2021. The effect of COVID-19 lockdowns on political support: Some good news for democracy? *European Journal of Political Research* 60: 497–505. [CrossRef]
Boin, Arjen, Paul't Hart, Eric Stern, and Bengt Sundelius. 2017. *The Politics of Crisis Management: Public Leadership under Pressure*. Cambridge: Cambridge University Press.
Boserup, Brad, Mark McKenney, and Adel Elkbuli. 2020. Alarming trends in US domestic violence during the COVID-19 pandemic. *The American Journal of Emergency Medicine* 38: 2753–55. [CrossRef] [PubMed]
Chan, K. H. Raymond. 2021. Tackling COVID-19 risk in Hong Kong: Examining distrust, compliance and risk management. *Current Sociology Monograph* 69: 547–65. [CrossRef]
Cole, Alistair, and Dionysios Stivas. 2020. Trust, Transparency and Transnational lessons from Covid 19. *Sage Advance*. Preprint. [CrossRef]
Cook, Karen S. 2001. *Trust in Society*. New York: Russel Sage Foundation.
Cucciniello, Maria, Gregory A. Porumbescu, and Stephan Grimmelikhuijsen. 2017. 25 Years of Transparency Research: Evidence and Future Directions. *Public Administration Review* 77: 32–44. [CrossRef]
Davis, Charles L. 1976. Social Mistrust as a Determinant of Political Cynicism in a Transitional Society: An Empirical Examination. *The Journal of Developing Areas* 11: 91–102.
Devine, Daniel, Jennifer Gaskell, and Will Jennings. 2020. Trust and the Coronavirus Pandemic: What are the Consequences of and for Trust? An Early Review of the Literature. *Political Studies Review* 19: 274–85. [CrossRef]
Diez Medrano, Juan. 1995. *La Opinión Pública Española y la Integración Europea: 1994 (Opiniones y Actitudes)*. Madrid: Centro de Investigaciones Sociológicas.
Downs, Timothy J., and Heidi J. Larson. 2007. Achieving Millennium Development Goals for Health: Building Understanding, Trust and Capacity to Respond. *Health Policy* 83: 144–61. [CrossRef]
Earle, Timothy C., and Michael Siegrist. 2008. Trust, Confidence and Cooperation model: A framework for understanding the relation between trust and Risk Perception. *International Journal Global Environmental Issues* 8: 17–29. [CrossRef]
Edelman. 2021. 2021 Edelman Trust Barometer Spring Update: A World in Trauma. Available online: https://www.edelman.com/trust/2021-trust-barometer/spring-update (accessed on 8 November 2021).
Fetzer, Thiemo, Marc Witte, Lukas Hensel, Jon M. Jachimowicz, Johannes Haushofer, Andriy Ivchenko, Stefano Caria, Elena Reutskaja, Christopher Roth, Stefano Fiorin, and et al. 2020. *Global Behaviors and Perceptions at the Onset of the COVID-19 Pandemic*. CAGE Online Working Paper Series 472; Swindon: Competitive Advantage in the Global Economy (CAGE).
Fisher, Justin, Jennifer van Heerde, and Andrew Tucker. 2010. Does on trust judgement fit? Linking theory and empirics. *British Journal of Politics and International Relations* 12: 161–88. [CrossRef]
Fledderus, Joost, Taco Branden, and Marlies Honingh. 2014. Restoring Trust Through the Co-Production of Public Services: A theoretical elaboration. *Public Management Review* 16: 424–43. [CrossRef]
Fraser, John. 1970. The Mistrustful-Efficacious Hypothesis and Political Participation. *The Journal of Politics* 32: 444–49. [CrossRef]
Grimmelikhuijsen, Stephan. 2012. Linking transparency, knowledge and citizen trust in government: An experiment. *International Review of Administrative Sciences* 78: 50–73. [CrossRef]
Groeniger, Joost Oude, Kjell Noordzij, Jeroen van der Waal, and Willem de Koster. 2021. Dutch COVID-19 lockdown measures increased trust in government and trust in science: A difference-in-difference analysis. *Social Science & Medicine* 275: 113819.
Hardin, Russell. 2002. *Trust and Trustworthiness*. New York: Russell Sage Foundation.
Heald, David. 2013. Varieties of Transparency. In *Transparency: The Key to Better Governance*. Edited by Hood Christopher and David Heald. Oxford: Oxford University Press, pp. 25–43.
Hilyard, Karen M., Vicki F. Freimuth, Donald Musa, Supriya Kumar, and Sandra Crouse Quinn. 2010. The Vagaries of Public Support for Government Actions in Case of a Pandemic. *Health Affairs* 29: 2294–301. [CrossRef]
Horvath, Agnes, Aprad Szakolczai, and Manussos Marangudakis. 2020. Modern Leaders. In *between Charisma and Trickery*. London: Routledge.
Huxtable, Richard. 2020. Covid-19: Where is the national ethical guidance? *BMC Medical Ethics* 21: 32. [CrossRef]

IPSOS. 2020. Coronavirus: Tracking UK Public Perception. Available online: https://www.ipsos.com/sites/default/files/2020--04/coronavirus-covid-19-infographic-ipsos-mori.pdf (accessed on 8 June 2021).
Keele, Luke. 2007. Social Capital and the Dynamics of Trust in Government. *American Journal of Political Science* 51: 241–54. [CrossRef]
Khosravi, Mohsen. 2020. Perceived risk of Covid-19 Pandemic: The Role of Public Worry and Trust. *Electronic Journal of General Medicine* 17: em203. [CrossRef]
Kruk, Margaret Elizabeth, and Lynn P. Freedman. 2008. Assessing health system performance in developing countries: A review of the literature. *Health Policy* 85: 263–76. [CrossRef]
Lanska, Douglas J. 1998. The Mad Cow Problem in the UK: Risk Perceptions, Risk Management, and Health Policy Development. *Journal of Public Health Policy* 19: 160–83. [CrossRef]
Lavazza, Andrea, and Mirko Farina. 2020. The role of experts in the COVID-19 pandemic and the limits of their epistemic authority in democracy. *Frontiers in Public Health* 8: 356. [CrossRef]
Lægreid, Per, and Lise H. Rykkja. 2019. *Societal Security and Crisis Management. Governance Capacity and Legitimacy*. Cham: Palgrave Macmillan.
Lo Yuk-ping, Catherine, and Nicholas Thomas. 2010. How is health a security issue? Politics, responses and issues. *Health Policy and Planning* 25: 447–53. [CrossRef]
Martin, Aaron, Andrea Carson, and Erik Baekkeskov. 2020. A Matter of Trust: Coronavirus Shows Again Why We Value Expertise When It Comes to Our Health. Available online: https://theconversation.com/a-matter-of-trust-coronavirus-shows-again-why-we-value-expertise-when-it-comes-to-our-health-134779 (accessed on 8 June 2021).
Meijer, Albert, Paul 't Hart, and Ben Worhty. 2018. Assessing government transparency: An interpretive framework. *Administration and Society* 50: 501–26. [CrossRef]
Newton, Kenneth. 2007. Social and Political Trust. In *The Oxford Handbook of Political Behaviour*. Edited by Russel J. Dalton and Hans-Dieter Klingemann. Oxford: Oxford University Press, pp. 342–61.
OECD. 2017. *Trust and Public Policy: How Better Governance Can Help Rebuild Public Trust*. Paris: OECD Publishing.
Oksanen, Atte, Markus Kaakinen, Rita Latikka, Iina Savolainen, Nina Savela, and Aki Koivula. 2020. Regulation and Trust: 3-Month Follow-up Study on COVID-19 Mortality in 25 European Countries. *JMIR Public Health and Surveillance* 6: e19218. [CrossRef]
Park, Heungsik, and John Blenkinsopp. 2011. The roles of transparency and trust in the relationship between corruption and citizen satisfaction. *International Review of Administrative Sciences* 77: 254–74. [CrossRef]
Parker, Suzanne L., Glenn R. Parker, and Terri L. Towner. 2014. Rethinking the Meaning and Measurement of Political Trust. In *Political Trust and Disenchantment with Politics International Perspectives*. Edited by Eder Christina, Ingvill C. Mochmann and Markus Quandt. Leiden: Brill, pp. 59–82.
PORI. 2021. People's Trust in the HKSAR Government. Available online: https://www.pori.hk/pop-poll/government-en/k001.html?lang=en (accessed on 8 November 2021).
Rieger, Marc Olivier, and Mei Wang. 2021. Trust in Government Actions During the COVID-19 Crisis. *Social Indicators Research*, 1–23. [CrossRef]
Rothstein, Bo. 2005. *Social Traps and Problems of Trust*. Cambridge: Cambridge University Press.
Rousseau, Denise M., Sim B. Sitkin, Ronald S. Burt, and Colin Camerer. 1998. Not so different after all: A cross-discipline view of trust. *Academy of Management Review* 23: 393–404. [CrossRef]
Rowe, Rosemary, and Michael Calnan. 2006. Trust relations in health care—The new agenda. *European Journal of Public Health* 16: 4–6. [CrossRef]
Seyd, Ben. 2020. Coronavirus: Trust in Political Figures Is at a Low Just as They Need Citizens to Act on Their Advice. Available online: https://theconversation.com/coronavirus-trust-in-political-figures-is-at-a-low-just-as-they-need-citizens-to-act-on-their-advice-133284 (accessed on 8 June 2021).
Shrank, William H., Teresa L. Rogstad, and Natasha Parekh. 2019. Waste in the US Health Care System: Estimated Costs and Potential for Savings. *The Journal of the American Medical Association* 322: 1501–9. [CrossRef]
Sibley, G. Chris, Lara M. Greaves, Nicole Satherley, Nickola C. Overall, Carol H.J. Lee, Petar Milojev, Joseph Bulbulia, Danny Osborne, Carla A. Houkamau, Marc S. Wilson, and et al. 2020. Effects of the COVID-19 pandemic and nationwide lockdown on trust, attitudes toward government, and well-being. *American Psychologist* 75: 618–30. [CrossRef]
Siegrist, Michael, and Alexandra Zingg. 2014. The role of public trust during pandemics. *European Psychologist* 19: 23–32. [CrossRef]
Sisk, Bryan, and Justin N. Baker. 2019. A Model of Interpersonal Trust, Credibility, and Relationship Maintenance. *Pediatrics* 144: e20191319. [CrossRef]
Slovic, Paul. 1999. Trust, emotion, sex, politics, and science: Surveying the risk-assessment battlefield. *Risk Analysis* 19: 689–701. [CrossRef] [PubMed]
Smith, Matthew. 2020. International COVID-19 Tracker Update: 18 May. *YouGov*. Available online: https://today.yougov.com/topics/international/articles-reports/2020/05/18/international-covid-19-tracker-update-18-may (accessed on 4 November 2021).
Stafford, Ian, Alistair Cole, and Dominic Heinz. 2022. *Analysing the Trust-Transparency Nexus: Multi-Level Governance in the UK, France and Germany*. Bristol: Policy Press, In print. ISBN 9781447355212.
Stafford, Ian. 2017. Measuring Trust and Transparency. Paper presented at 24th International Conference of Europeanists, Glasgow, UK, July 12–14.
Sztompka, Piotr. 2006. New Perspectives on Trust. *American Journal of Sociology* 112: 905–19. [CrossRef]

van de Walle, Steven, and Alasdair Roberts. 2008. Publishing performance information: An illusion of control? In *Performance Information in the Public Sector: How It Is Used*. Edited by Wooter van Dooren and Steven van de Walle. Basingstoke: Palgrave, pp. 211–26.

van der Meer, Tom, and Armen Hakhverdian. 2017. Political Trust as the Evaluation of Process and Performance: A Cross-National Study of 42 European Countries. *Political Studies* 65: 81–102. [CrossRef]

van der Weerd, Willemien, Danielle Rm Timmermans, Desiree Jma Beaujean, Jurriaan Oyudhoff, and Jim E. van Steenbergen. 2011. Monitoring the level of government trust, risk perception and intention of the general public to adopt protective measures during the influenza A (H1N1) pandemic in the Netherlands. *BMC Public Health* 11: 575. [CrossRef] [PubMed]

Veillard, Jeremy, F. Champagne, N. Klazinga, V. Kazandjian, O.A. Arah, and A.-L. Guisset. 2005. A performance assessment framework for hospitals: The WHO regional office for Europe PATH project. *International Journal for Quality in Health Care* 17: 487–96. [CrossRef]

YouGov. 2021. COVID-19: Government Handling and Confidence in Health Authorities. Available online: https://yougov.co.uk/topics/international/articles-reports/2020/03/17/perception-government-handling-covid-19 (accessed on 8 November 2021).

Zhu, Viviana. 2020. Fighting the Coronavirus Pandemic, East Asian Responses—Hong Kong: Border Management, Epidemiological Tracking and Social Responsibility. Available online: https://www.institutmontaigne.org/en/blog/fighting-coronavirus-pandemic-east-asian-responses-hong-kong-border-management-epidemiological (accessed on 8 June 2021).

Zmerli, Sonja, and Ken Newton. 2011. Winners, Losers and Three Types of Trust. In *Political Trust: Why Context Matters*. Edited by Sonja Zmerli and Marc Hooghe. Colchester: ECPR Press, pp. 67–94.

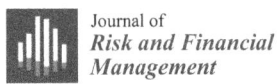

Article

The COVID-19 Health Crisis and Its Impact on China's International Relations

Jean-Pierre Cabestan

Department of Government and International Studies, Hong Kong Baptist University, Kowloon, Hong Kong, China; cabestan@hkbu.edu.hk

Abstract: Using qualitative methods, this article focuses on the relationship between the COVID-19 health crisis and China's foreign policy and foreign relations. My main argument is that since its outbreak in late 2019, the COVID-19 health crisis has deepened the tensions already existing between China and the United States, as well as China and the West in general. Other factors that appeared before the pandemic have also contributed to intensifying the Sino-US rivalry as well as Sino-European frictions. Nonetheless, Beijing's proactive mask and vaccine diplomacy, its strict lockdown policy as well as its more aggressive nationalist and anti-western narrative have fed rather than alleviated these tensions. While China's image in the Global South has remained largely positive, in the Global North, it has rapidly deteriorated. All in all, this paper demonstrates that the pandemic has been an aggravating factor contributing to the downward spiral of China's relations with the outside world as well as its own isolation.

Keywords: COVID-19; China; United States; European Union; Xi Jinping; Donald Trump; Joe Biden

Citation: Cabestan, Jean-Pierre. 2022. The COVID-19 Health Crisis and Its Impact on China's International Relations. *Journal of Risk and Financial Management* 15: 123. https://doi.org/10.3390/jrfm15030123

Academic Editor: Thanasis Stengos

Received: 10 January 2022
Accepted: 3 March 2022
Published: 4 March 2022

Publisher's Note: MDPI stays neutral with regard to jurisdictional claims in published maps and institutional affiliations.

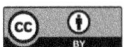

Copyright: © 2022 by the author. Licensee MDPI, Basel, Switzerland. This article is an open access article distributed under the terms and conditions of the Creative Commons Attribution (CC BY) license (https://creativecommons.org/licenses/by/4.0/).

1. Introduction

To what extent has the COVID-19 health crisis influenced and changed China's foreign policy and international role? To what extent has it affected China's relations with the United States and the European Union (EU)? How has it influenced China's relations with the Global South? These are the questions that this article ambitions to briefly address. These questions relate both to China's international policies and actions as well as outside perceptions of and reactions to these policies and actions.

To be sure, many of China's policies and actions (e.g., its assertiveness and competition with the US (and the West)) predate the pandemic. Nonetheless, my hypothesis is that the pandemic has highlighted and enhanced China's assertiveness as well as intensified this competition. Instead of fostering cooperation as some, including the Chinese government, had hoped (*Xinhua* 2020b), COVID-19 has fed frictions and tensions between China and developed democracies. At the same time, COVID-19 has contributed to increasing China's influence in the Global South in spite of several cases of pushback which the West has managed to capitalize upon.

Not many articles have been published on this issue. I contributed a study in the early phase of the crisis (Cabestan 2020a). Among the other analyses, some have questioned or minimized the impact of the pandemic on Chinese foreign policy (Raman and Murkherjee 2021) and more broadly the world order (Nye 2020). As we will see, I do not completely disagree with this view, although I do think that COVID-19 aggravated the situation. Aside from that, works that speculated that China would use the pandemic to assert its ambition to change international norms have made the right prediction (Haenle 2020).

This article adopts a neo-realist approach of international relations inspired by Randall Schweller (2006). While it recognizes the structural nature of the Sino-US geo-strategic rivalry, it also takes into account the influence of domestic factors, particularly of the political and ideological differences between both powers' polities. Yet, it also factors in perceptions and misperceptions, to use a concept promoted by Robert Jervis (1976), and how nationalism has strengthened their impact on policies.

Using qualitative methods, this article attempts to isolate the pandemic factor and assess its weight and impact on China's foreign policy and foreign relations. While it covers a short period of time, which started in late 2019 after the new coronavirus was discovered in Wuhan, it also puts back the emergence of the pandemic in the broader context of growing competition between China and the United States and China and the West in general. This article is divided into four sections: the first one briefly presents China's growing international ambitions prior to the outbreak of the pandemic; the second one analyzes China's COVID-19 diplomacy and its "overkill" dimension; the third one evaluates the impact of COVID-19 Chinese activism on its relations with the north, especially the United States and the European Union; and the final section assesses the impact of China's COVID-19 diplomacy on its relations with the Global South.

2. China's International Role before COVID-19

To better isolate COVID-19 and assess its impact, it is necessary to briefly revisit and present China's growing international role before the pandemic erupted in late 2019 and became a pandemic in the following spring. Since Xi Jinping became General Secretary of the Chinese Communist Party (CCP) in late 2012 and before 2020, China had already more clearly asserted its foreign policy posture. As a result, its relationship with the United States became more contentious, and with the European Union, it became more complicated.

2.1. A More Assertive Foreign and Security Policy

It can be argued that this assertiveness goes back to 2008, the Beijing Olympics and the international financial crisis. Then, the Chinese government started to feel that the West, and particularly the United States, were in decline, opening wider China's window of strategic opportunity. Yet, it was Xi, not his predecessor Hu Jintao, who abandoned for good Deng Xiaoping's low-profile diplomacy (韜光養晦 *daoguang yanghui*) and replaced it with a much more proactive and assertive foreign policy, encapsulated in the slogan "strives for achievements" (奮發有為 *fenfa youwei*) (Doshi 2021a).

There was no coincidence that it was around the same time in the autumn of 2013 that Xi announced the launching of the new land (one belt) and maritime (one road) silk roads, or "one belt, one road" (OBOR, 一帶一路 *yidai yilu*), a policy that was 2 years later renamed in English the "Belt and Road Initiative" (BRI). Aimed at intensifying China's economic connectivity with and as a result their footprint in the world, the BRI mainly enhanced its loans and investments in infrastructure projects in the Global South (Zhao 2020).

Since 2012 as well, Beijing has started to become more assertive in the maritime domain that it claims and within what is called the "first island chain", a string of islands which goes all the way from Okinawa to Borneo via Taiwan and the Philippines. In the South China Sea, after having annexed Scarborough Shoal in April 2012, a land feature long occupied by Manila and located 200 km west of Luzon, the Chinese government started to build artificial islands on the rocks that it had controlled since the late 1980s in the Spratlys and later militarized them (Hayton 2014; Shambaugh 2020). In the East China Sea, Chinese coast guard ships increased their intrusions in the contiguous and territorial waters around the Senkaku (or Diaoyu), a group of small islands administered by Japan since 1895 and claimed by China and Taiwan since the early 1970s (O'Hanlon 2019).

That aside, after Ms. Tsai Ing-wen's election as president of Taiwan and the return of the independence-leaning Democratic Progressive Party (DPP) to power, Xi has adopted a much more aggressive posture toward the island state, indicating a clear intention to not only refuse any contact with the new Taiwanese authorities as long as they do not endorse the "one China principle" but also to speed up unification with the mainland by any means, including the use of force and the implementation of the "one country, two systems" formula in the island (Cole 2020).

This more ambitious foreign and security policy was confirmed by Xi in his report to the 19th CCP Congress in 2017. Now, China is "moving towards the world's central stage" and hopes to become a full-fledged military great power by 2049, the occasion of the 100th anniversary of the People's Republic of China, capable of supplanting the United States, including militarily, and as a result replacing it as the world's top superpower (Xi 2017).

In order to achieve these new objectives, the Chinese government has introduced a more proactive but also aggressive foreign policy posture, often referred to as "Wolf Warrior diplomacy" (戰狼外交 *zhanlang waijiao*). This expression was inspired by the successful 2017 Chinese movie titled *Wolf Warrior 2*, which describes how China is now able to protect its interests and nationals overseas, especially in civil war-torn African countries (Martin 2021).

2.2. A Growing Rivalry with the US

China's new objectives and ambitions could only trigger a more intense rivalry with the United States. While president Obama had already decided to "pivot" to Asia as early as 2011, the US rebalancing became more decisive under his successor Donald Trump. In the meantime, introducing in 2015 its "Made in China 2025" strategy, Beijing had shown a clear intention to catch up with America on the technological front. In the same period, spurred by the BRI, US-China competition had intensified in the Global South, in Southeast Asia, in Africa, in the Middle East, in Latin America and even in the South Pacific (Breslin 2021). In the same period of time, the People's Liberation Army (PLA) sped up its modernization, particularly the expansion of its navy. Additionally, in 2017, it opened its first naval base overseas in Djibouti, a strategic chokepoint situated in the Horn of Africa and next to the Bab-el-Mandeb and the Gulf of Aden (Cabestan 2020b).

The launching of the US-China trade war in the spring of 2018 has been the most visible and publicized feature of this growing rivalry. However, far from being only commercial, this competition has also rapidly appeared to be both geostrategic and ideological. In 2019, the Trump administration adopted a new Indo-Pacific strategy openly aimed at better balancing, or some would say "containing", China's growing diplomatic and military ambitions in the region. At the same time, the Quad, the quadrilateral security dialogue among the US, Japan, India and Australia, was revived and strengthened. Although the Trump Administration did not initially give much attention to human rights issues, the deterioration of the situation in Hong Kong after the failure of the 2019 protest movement and in Xinjiang, where more than 1 million Uighurs had been detained without trial, forced it to react, and this was before the COVID pandemic broke out (Pillsbury 2020).

2.3. A More Complicated Relationship with the European Union

Prior to COVID, EU-China relations had already become more difficult. In March 2019, the EU Commission had stated that "China is, simultaneously, in different policy areas, a cooperation partner with whom the EU has closely aligned objectives, a negotiating partner with whom the EU needs to find a balance of interests, an economic competitor in the pursuit of technological leadership, and a systemic rival promoting alternative models of governance" (European Commission 2019). The number of irritants had obviously increased, including the lack of market access of EU companies in China, the forced technology transfers imposed on them when they invest in China, the subsidies provided by the Chinese government to its companies, especially its state-owned enterprises (SOEs), in spite of its commitments to the WTO rules, Beijing's promotion of 16 + 1 (17 after Greece joined in 2019 and 16 again after Lithuania left in 2021), a forum bringing Central and Eastern countries together every year, including 12 (now 11) EU member-states, and China and promoting business and investment relations with the help of the BRI, as well as human rights issues, a bone of contention which had become more serious as the Xi government intensified its crackdowns of dissidents, activists and autonomy defenders in Tibet, Xinjiang and later in Hong Kong (Godement 2020).

3. China's COVID-19 Diplomacy: Overkill

When the health crisis turned into a pandemic, China became hyperactive on the international stage, strongly defending its own behavior and strategy (Xinhua 2020b). However, it ambitioned to achieve too many objectives at the same time, both trying to appear as a generous country and manifesting an offensive nationalism. As a result, Beijing's "overkill" boomeranged, feeding the existing tensions and contributing to isolating China (Cabestan 2020a).

3.1. China's Defensive and Offensive Strategies

On the one hand, the Chinese authorities pursued defensive objectives. The coronavirus originated in Wuhan in December 2019, but until 23 January 2020, when Xi Jinping decided to execute a national lockdown, they tried to hide the existence of a pandemic and let its citizens travel abroad, facilitating the dissemination of the virus. In contrast, after 23 January, China's behavior changed 180 degrees; it closed the country from the outside and imposed strict quarantine measures on all travelers.

At the same time, Beijing embarked on proactive COVID diplomacy, providing large quantities of masks and PPE (personnel protective equipment) to a large number of countries both in the Global North and the Global South. However, that was not all. To better defend its own policy, the Chinese government minimized the assistance that it first received from other countries (e.g., the EU) and launched a disinformation campaign about the origin of the virus, propagating the idea that some American army athletes had transmitted it to Chinese counterparts in the international military games organized in Wuhan in October 2019 (Cabestan 2020a).

On the other hand, the Chinese government adopted an offensive strategy, trying hard to appear as a responsible great power and a model member of the international community, in particular to the World Health Organization (WHO) (Xinhua 2020a). It promoted the idea that China was a "model" in terms of health crisis management, capitalizing on the difficulties encountered by other countries, particularly democracies, and boasting about the efficiency of its CCP-led system of governance. More generally, the Chinese propaganda apparatus took advantage of the COVID crisis to intensify its nationalist discourse, with the intention to both glue the society around the government and sell China's success story around the world (Zhao 2022). In the WHO as well, it worked hard to be perceived as a model participant in the global fight against the pandemic, and this was despite an attempt to manipulate the organization leadership as well as a reluctance to provide timely information to the WHO and let WHO experts investigate in China, especially in Wuhan. For example, Beijing put pressure on WHO Director General Tedros Adhanom Ghebreyesus to postpone until 30 January its decision to declare COVID-19 a public health emergency of international concern (PHEIC) and until 11 March to elevate it to the status of pandemic, slowing down any global or country-based measures to stop it.

In other words, spurred by a growing nationalism at home that they stimulated on purpose, the Chinese authorities have attempted to reach too many objectives at the same time, compromising the efficiency of both their message and their action.

3.2. The Impact of China's COVID Strategy on Its Relations with the World

Rapidly, criticism of China's behavior vis-à-vis the pandemic emerged in the world, first in the developed countries and also in the Global South.

Beijing's criticism of the Trump administration's early decision, made in late January 2020, to stop air traffic with China did not go over well in the United States, all the more because, not long after, the Chinese authorities did the same and in a more forceful manner. However, it was the latter's attempt to control the WHO's COVID discourse and strategy that triggered the US' fiercest criticism. A former Ethiopian Health Minister, Tedros was himself attacked for being too close and obedient to China, which took advantage of this inclination as well as the opacity of its own health system to impose its own approach on the WHO (Feldwisch-Drentrup 2020). Since the WHO is a rather weak multilateral organization which is traditionally highly dependent upon the cooperation of the country where the epidemy originates from, the Chinese government easily achieved its objective. For example, Beijing managed to ban worldwide any reference to the "Wuhan flu" and instead call the new pandemic COVID-19.

Moreover, China's lack of transparency and limits imposed on any WHO investigation team fed suspicions about the veracity of the data that it publicized. Officially, only around 130,000 Chinese people got COVID, and less than 5000 of them subsequently died of COVID (130,398 and 4824, respectively, by 25 February 2022) (BBC 2022). However, reports published in the US in 2020 already indicated much higher figures—probably up to 2.9 million cases and tens of thousands of deaths—even if these data show that China managed to keep the virus under control much faster than many other countries (Scissors 2020). More recent studies have made Chinese official data even less credible (Calhoun 2022a, 2022b).

Another criticism had to do with the quality of the equipment delivered by China and the fact that the Chinese government mixed up aid with sales, blurring the distinction between the two and propagating the false impression that it was more generous than any other nation (ChinaPower 2021).

More generally, China's Wolf Warrior diplomacy and anti-western discourse have led to a battle of narratives with many countries (Sun 2020). This has included the European Union and, in particular, France. There, the Chinese Ambassador Lu Shaye was summoned to the French Foreign Ministry in April 2020 for having disseminated on the Embassy's website inaccurate information about the lack of attention given to COVID patients in some French hospitals (Huang 2021).

A more unexpected development took place around the same time in Canton (Guangzhou), where cases of racial discrimination emerged; a number of Africans had been expelled from their flats, their landlord fearing that they were contaminated with COVID. This triggered strong reactions from the public opinion and even the government in several African countries, especially Nigeria, forcing the Chinese Foreign Ministry to go out of its way to mend relations with them (Ngcobo 2021).

Another issue that the pandemic has exacerbated has been developing countries' growing debt. To be sure, far from all their debt is due to China. In June 2020, Beijing endorsed the debt relief plan known as the "G20 Debt Service Suspension Initiative" (DSSI) adopted by the G20 meeting held that month. Then, it announced the suspension of debt repayment for 77 developing countries, as well as a financial help of USD 2 billion over 2 years for countries hit by the coronavirus pandemic (*Global Times* 2020). Later however, the Chinese government clearly showed a preference for rescheduling debt repayments rather than granting debt forgiveness, affecting its image in the Global South and particularly in Africa (see below).

The final question was the fierce competition for vaccines' R&D and international distribution. Instead of mitigating tensions among great powers, this competition has intensified them. China offered its own emergency vaccines to many developing countries even before they had been approved by the WHO, triggering suspicion about their safety and efficacy among the recipient countries. Later, Beijing joined the WHO's sponsored COVAX distribution scheme, competing with the US and Europe to appear as a key player in vaccine donations (see below).

All in all, China's COVID activism and nationalism have had mixed results. While its mask, PPE and vaccine diplomacy may have consolidated China's position in some developing countries, overall, it has contributed to deteriorating its image and underscoring a growing rivalry with the West and not only the United States.

4. China's Post-Pandemic International Activism and Changing Perception of China

China's deteriorating image in the West and part of the Global South has not stopped its ambition to play a bigger role on the international stage. On the contrary, its ability to get out of the pandemic and to resume normal economic activities as soon as in the second half of 2020 and consequently ahead of most countries convinced the Beijing authorities that they could take advantage of this new situation to push their envelope and become even more self-confident and proactive.

As a result, they intensified their anti-Western discourse and diplomacy. While it started to be mentioned in 2017, "the East is rising the West is declining" (東升西降 *donsheng xijiang*) as a slogan became much more quoted both by the CCP propaganda and Chinese international relations experts (Doshi 2021b). This new discourse has been more successful in the Global South than in the "Global North".

4.1. China's Post-Pandemic International Activism

First of all, since it approved its first homemade vaccine (Sinopharm) in December 2020, China has developed proactive vaccine diplomacy, especially in poor countries. There, it is a major player today. In May 2021, Sinopharm became the first Chinese vaccine endorsed by the WHO. This was followed a month later by CoronaVac, manufactured by Sinovac. As a result, in October 2021, both Chinese vaccines counted for almost half of all the COVID-19 vaccines distributed globally, with CoronaVac being the most frequently used vaccine in the world today ahead of Pfiser-BioNTech (Mallapaty 2021). True, their efficacy may be lower (79% and 51%, respectively, against over 90% for BioNTech). Nonetheless, in early August 2021, China claimed to have already supplied many more doses (750 million against 110 million for the US) to developing countries than others (104 against 65) (Leng and Hu 2021). These recipients included a lot of BRI nations.

This distribution effort, however, has been far from free. Among the 1.3 billion doses distributed by China by early October 2021, an estimated 71.9 million doses, or 5.5%, had been donated. True, China was ahead of the US, which announced only in May 2021 the distribution of 80 million doses free of charge worldwide. However, the perception that China was selling rather than donating vaccines compelled the Chinese government to adjust its policy. In September 2021, Xi Jinping pledged that China would donate 100 million COVID-19 vaccine doses to developing countries by the end of this year (Ma 2021). In November 2021, at the 8th Forum of China Africa Cooperation (FOCAC) in Dakar, Xi promised to provide 1 billion doses of vaccines to Africa, including 600 million doses as a donation (*Xinhua* 2021a). Still, 40% of the Chinese vaccines distributed to Africa will be sold rather than donated.

The other issue for which China also adjusted (to some extent) its policy is debt relief and rescheduling. In 2020–2021, Chinese lenders provided USD 12.1 billion in global debt relief, including USD 1.3 billion under the G20 DSSI relief program. However, by July 2021, the amount of interest-free loan debts cancelled remained small—USD 114 million to 15 African countries—against repayment deferrals amounting to around USD 7 billion, mainly in favor of Angola (USD 6.2 billion) and Ecuador (USD 891 million) (China Africa Research Initiative (CARI) 2021).

Beyond COVID-19 and the debt crisis, China wants more than ever to be seen both as the leader of the South and the world's "silent majority", providing a new and better model of governance to the world. To that end, Beijing has continued to invest in the United Nations system, enhancing its influence in it and convincing several of its agencies to adopt Xi Jinping's formula about the "common future of mankind". More broadly, the Chinese Communist Party has intensified its ideological rivalry with the West, promoting its own political system as "a democracy that works" in opposition to American and more generally Western democracies which are, in its eyes, unable to deliver good and efficient governance (*Xinhua* 2021b).

4.2. China's Contrasted Image in the World

China's post-COVID-19 international activism has had a contrasting impact. While its image has clearly deteriorated in the North, it has overall remained strong in the Global South.

In October 2020, according to the Pew Center Survey (Silver et al. 2020), unfavorable views of China had reached "historic highs" in many countries. Across the 14 nations surveyed, a median of 61% thought that China had done a bad job dealing with the COVID-19 outbreak. This was many more than those who said the same of the way the pandemic had been handled by their own country, by the WHO or by the EU (except the US (84%)), Japan (79%), Australia (73%), France (54%) or Italy (49%).

In June 2021, while US's image had recovered (61% favorable view), China's image has remained largely negative among developed countries (27% favorable view) (Silver 2021).

The limit of these surveys is obvious: only developed countries were included.

If we look at Afrobarometer data for example, China's image may have gone down a bit compared to pre-COVID times, but favorable views about this country's influence in Africa remained largely positive (60% in 2020 against 65% in 2015). This does not mean the Africans' view of the US has deteriorated; it has remained rather strong (58%) ahead of the former colonial powers (46%) or Russia (38%). However, rather than opposing both great powers, as many developing countries' citizens, Africans that "feel positively about the influence of China are more likely to hold positive view of the US influence" (Sheehy and Asunka 2021).

Yet, in closing its borders for over 2 years, China complicated its relations with many countries, especially the Asian part of the world, which has close economic relations with it (Wang 2021; Yang 2022).

5. COVID-19 Pandemic Impact on China-Global North Relations

China's activism both after the outbreak of the pandemic and in the post-pandemic period has had a very negative impact on its relations with the Global North. The United States under Trump, and later under Biden, has adopted a much more confrontational strategy toward China. While the EU has been slower to adjust, its China policy has also evolved toward a more critical and robust posture.

5.1. Impact on China-US Relations

By and large, the COVID-19 pandemic has contributed to deepening the Sino-US rivalry. More visible at the end of the Trump presidency, this rivalry has intensified under Biden. Of course, as we will see, other factors have played a role. Among them, the repression of the 2019 protest movement and the introduction of a National Security Law in June 2020 in Hong Kong need to be mentioned. These developments convinced Secretary of State Mike Pompeo to push later that year for a regime change in China. However, China's more assertive posture has united the Americans in their intention to push back. Consequently, the Biden administration has largely carried on Trump's China policy. The trade war has gone on, even if the original intention to "decouple" with the Chinese economy has been abandoned. In September 2021, together with Australia and the United Kingdom, the US concluded a new pact, AUKUS, whose objective is also to rein in China's aggressive military plans, especially vis-à-vis Taiwan and in the South China Sea. Aside from that, on human rights, while Biden has become more subdued on the regime change issue, he has increased his government's pressure as well as the ideological battle between authoritarian China and democracies (Manning 2021).

Yet, the way the Chinese authorities have handled the health crisis has been an aggravating factor in the deterioration of China-US relations. For example, as early as January 2020, the Trump administration accused that Chinese leaders "intentionally concealed the severity" of the pandemic from the world. This was followed by a battle of narratives about the origins of the virus which added to the tensions between both countries (Council on Foreign Relations 2021).

With Biden, some hoped that Sino-American cooperation on the pandemic at least would take shape, but this has not been the case. After the Biden administration re-joined the WHO, both powers deepened their competition both in terms of vaccine distribution and debt relief. While the US has been slow to provide vaccines and assistance, it has been catching up with the firm intention to not let China dominate the game. More generally, the pandemic has accelerated the US plan to reorganize supply chains and reduce its dependence upon China and not only as far as masks, PPEs or vaccines are concerned.

All in all, the pandemic has consolidated a US-China geo-strategic rivalry. Since this rivalry is structural, the result has not been surprising (deLisle 2021).

5.2. Impact on China-EU Relations

The EU and EU member states have been slower to react. The growing dissatisfaction of European public opinion with China did not prevent the EU from negotiating and approving in principle the Comprehensive Accord on Investment (CAI) with China in December 2020. Here again, other factors, especially the increasingly worrisome human rights situation in Xinjiang and Hong Kong, have played their part in the deterioration of Sino-European relations. For the first time in its history, in March 2021, the EU imposed targeted sanctions on a few Chinese officials in charge of Xinjiang, triggering Beijing's decision to launch a series of countersanctions against a few European activists, including members of the EU Parliament who had been critical of China. This latter decision has contributed to compromising any endorsement of the CAI by the EU Parliament, leaving it in limbo in the foreseeable future.

Nonetheless, China's handling of the pandemic has accelerated the deterioration of Sino-EU relations. Meanwhile, in spite of COVID and the growing Sino-US tensions, some EU countries such as Hungary or non-EU nations such as Serbia have maintained a good relationship with China, and spurred by a more critical public opinion, the EU mainstream view about China has changed (Seaman 2020). Less naiveté and more realism were already perceptible in the EU China policy in the summer of 2020 (Le Corre and Brattberg 2020). However, more recently, the EU's attitude toward China has not been more accommodating in spite of Xi Jinping' repeated effort to drive a wedge between Europeans and Americans and US clumsiness toward France in the preparation and announcement of the AUKUS pact (Ganster 2021). As with the US, the EU wants to continue its dialogue and cooperation with China on many issues, including of course climate change (Emmott 2021), but the pandemic has helped the EU realize the true ambitions of China not only in its neighborhood, especially vis-à-vis Taiwan, but also in the world. In other words, competition has clearly taken the lead over cooperation.

6. Conclusions

Using qualitative methods as well as surveys, this article has demonstrated that the COVID-19 health crisis has been an aggravating factor, contributing to making both China's foreign policy more assertive and its relations with the outside world, especially its major partners, more contentious. Having gotten out of the health crisis and its domestic lockdown (with a few local exceptions) faster and having fewer cases than any other large country, China has good reason to feel stronger today. As a result, it has no reasons to change course. The successful organization of the Beijing Winter Olympics in February 2022 and the long Sino-Russian joint statement issued on the day of its opening ceremony, which President Vladimir Putin attended, are perfect illustrations of China's and Xi Jinping's self-confidence and ambition to change the world order (Yu 2022). True, the pandemic has not fundamentally changed China's foreign policy and its relations with its major partners, nor it has really changed the world order. In that sense, I agree with other analyses presented above (Nye 2020; Raman and Murkherjee 2021). As this article has also shown, today's trends in Chinese foreign policy were already at play before. Nevertheless, the pandemic has intensified tensions and irritants, deteriorating China's image, especially in the North (except in Russia), and accelerating the readjustment of US's and later EU's own China policy. While geostrategic realities and differences of political values laid the groundwork for COVID-19 to become a source of contention (Schweller 2006), perceptions both in China and outside of China have played a role (Jervis 1976).

The pandemic has given an opportunity for China to reach out to more countries as well as enhance its cooperation with them within the WHO (COVAX) or bilaterally. Its image in the Global South has gone down a bit, but it has remained largely positive.

Taking advantage of the BRI, China's diplomatic activism has directly helped maintain this overall good perception. However, at the same time, the COVID-19 pandemic has slowed down China's interactions with the rest of the world, contributing to isolating the country from the international community. Xi Jinping has not left China since January 2020 and has met a handful of foreign official guests since then. Most other leaders, such as Prime Minister Li Keqiang, have not traveled abroad either, leaving this job to the two most senior officials in charge of foreign affairs, Politburo member Yang Jiechi and Foreign Minister (and State Councilor) Wang Yi. Overall, justified by the quarantine restrictions imposed on any large Chinese delegation traveling abroad, this deliberate decision to reduce to a trickle high-level contacts with the outside world has been detrimental to China, both for its image and the credibility of its foreign policy, and the organization of more frequent visioconferences with other heads of state or government could not really replace face-to-face meetings. The surge of new COVID-19 variants, such as Omicron, has been conducive to keeping many of China's doors closed, feeding distrust with the rest of the world, particularly the Global North.

More broadly, the COVID-19 health crisis has intensified China's competition with the Global North. Instead of bringing together nations to fight against a common evil, such as the battle against climate change arguably succeeded in doing in Glasgow in November 2021 (COP26), the pandemic has contributed to making competition prevail even more over cooperation in the context of a growing rivalry and perhaps a new Cold War between China and the US and, more broadly, China and the West.

Funding: This research was funded by the Hung Hin Shiu Charitable Foundation, by the Hong Kong Baptist University Research Committee (Project 165234) and by the Heinrich Boell Stiftung.

Institutional Review Board Statement: Not applicable.

Informed Consent Statement: Not applicable.

Data Availability Statement: Not applicable.

Conflicts of Interest: The authors declare no conflict of interest.

References

BBC. 2022. COVID Map: Coronavirus Cases, Deaths, Vaccinations by Country. Available online: https://www.bbc.com/news/world-51235105 (accessed on 25 February 2022).

Breslin, Shaun. 2021. *China Risen. Studying Chinese Global Power*. Bristol: Bristol University Press.

Cabestan, Jean-Pierre. 2020a. China's Battle with Coronavirus: Possible Geopolitical Gains and Real Challenges. *Reports, Al Jazeera Center for Studies*, April 19. Available online: https://studies.aljazeera.net/en/reports/china%E2%80%99s-battle-coronavirus-possible-geopolitical-gains-and-real-challenges (accessed on 25 February 2022).

Cabestan, Jean-Pierre. 2020b. China's Military Base in Djibouti: A Microcosm of China's Growing Competition with the United States and New Bipolarity. *Journal of Contemporary China* 29: 731–47. [CrossRef]

Calhoun, George. 2022a. Beijing Is Intentionally Underreporting China's COVID Death Rate. Part 1. *Forbes*, January 2. Available online: https://www.forbes.com/sites/georgecalhoun/2022/01/02/beijing-is-intentionally-underreporting-chinas-COVID-death-rate-part-1/?sh=2bf3ea394352 (accessed on 25 February 2022).

Calhoun, George. 2022b. Beijing Is Intentionally Underreporting China's COVID Death Rate. Part II. *Forbes*, January 5. Available online: https://www.forbes.com/sites/georgecalhoun/2022/01/05/beijing-is-intentionally-underreporting-chinas-COVID-death-rate-part-2/?sh=34655c3873b8 (accessed on 2 February 2022).

China Africa Research Initiative (CARI). 2021. Global Debt Relief Dashboard. Johns Hopkins School of Advanced International Studies. Available online: http://www.sais-cari.org/debt-relief (accessed on 25 February 2022).

ChinaPower. 2021. *Is China COVID-19 Diplomacy Succeeding?* Washington, DC: CSIS, September 7, Available online: https://chinapower.csis.org/china-COVID-medical-vaccine-diplomacy/ (accessed on 25 February 2022).

Cole, J. Michael. 2020. *Cross-Strait Relations Since 2016: The End of the Illusion*. London and New York: Routledge.

Council on Foreign Relations. 2021. The Origins of COVID-19: Implications for U.S.-China Relations. *Meeting*, July 13. Available online: https://www.cfr.org/event/origins-COVID-19-implications-us-china-relations (accessed on 25 February 2022).

deLisle, Jacques. 2021. When Rivalry Goes Viral: COVID-19, U.S.-China Relations, and East Asia. *Orbis* 65: 46–74. [CrossRef]

Doshi, Rush. 2021a. *The Long Game: China's Grand Strategy to Displace American Order*. Oxford: Oxford University Press.
Doshi, Rush. 2021b. Great Changes Unseen in a Century: The Elusive Phrase Driving China's Grand Strategy. *China Leadership Monitor*, June 1. Available online: https://3c8314d6-0996-4a21-9f8a-a63a59b09269.filesusr.com/ugd/af1ede_c6526da05ad84ddcba3a8ce4b1c6d8f1.pdf (accessed on 25 February 2022).
Emmott, Robin. 2021. EU, China Agree to Hold Summit, Michel Says after Xi Call. *Reuters*, October 15. Available online: https://www.reuters.com/world/europe/eu-china-agree-hold-summit-michel-says-after-xi-call-2021-10-15/ (accessed on 26 January 2022).
European Commission. 2019. EU-China—A Strategic Outlook. Joint Communication to the European Parliament, the European Council and the Council. March 12. Available online: https://ec.europa.eu/info/sites/default/files/communication-eu-china-a-strategic-outlook.pdf (accessed on 26 January 2022).
Feldwisch-Drentrup, Hinnerk. 2020. How WHO Became China's Coronavirus Accomplice. *Foreign Policy*, April 2. Available online: https://foreignpolicy.com/2020/04/02/china-coronavirus-who-health-soft-power/ (accessed on 26 January 2022).
Ganster, Ronja. 2021. Post-Pademic EU-China Relations: Navigating Rough Waters in Unprecedented Times. *European Student Think Tank*, March 27. Available online: https://esthinktank.com/2021/03/27/post-pandemic-eu-china-relations-navigating-rough-waters-in-unprecedented-times/ (accessed on 26 January 2022).
Global Times. 2020. China Suspends Debt Repayment for 77 Developing Nations, Regions. *Global Times*, June 7. Available online: https://www.globaltimes.cn/content/1190790.shtml (accessed on 25 February 2022).
Godement, François. 2020. *Europe's Pushback on China*. Policy Paper. Paris: Institut Montaigne, Available online: https://www.institutmontaigne.org/ressources/pdfs/publications/europes-pushback-china-intention-policy-paper.pdf (accessed on 26 January 2022).
Haenle, Paul. 2020. What the Coronavirus Mean for China's Foreign Policy? Carnegie Endowment for International Peace. *Q&A*, March 11. Available online: https://carnegieendowment.org/2020/03/11/what-coronavirus-means-for-china-s-foreign-policy-pub-81259 (accessed on 25 February 2022).
Hayton, Bill. 2014. *The South China Sea. The Struggle for Power in Asia*. New Haven: Yale University Press.
Huang, Zhao Alexandre. 2021. "Wolf Warrior" and China's digital public diplomacy during the COVID-19 crisis. *Place Branding and Public Policy*, October 26. Available online: https://link.springer.com/article/10.1057/s41254-021-00241-3 (accessed on 24 January 2022).
Jervis, Robert. 1976. *Perceptions and Misperceptions in International Relations*. Princeton: Princeton University Press.
Le Corre, Philippe, and Erik Brattberg. 2020. How the Coronavirus Pandemic Shattered Europe's Illusions of China. *Carnegie Endowment for International Peace*, July 9. Available online: https://carnegieendowment.org/2020/07/09/how-coronavirus-pandemic-shattered-europe-s-illusions-of-china-pub-82265 (accessed on 24 January 2022).
Leng, Shumei, and Yuwei Hu. 2021. China to Provide 2 Billion Doses of Vaccine to World This Year. *Global Times*, August 5. Available online: https://www.globaltimes.cn/page/202108/1230714.shtml (accessed on 24 January 2022).
Ma, Josephine. 2021. US-China Coronavirus Vaccine Diplomacy Heats Up but Can Donations Sway Allegiances? *South China Morning Post*. October 13. Available online: https://www.scmp.com/news/china/diplomacy/article/3152098/us-china-coronavirus-vaccine-diplomacy-heats-can-donations (accessed on 25 January 2022).
Mallapaty, Smriti. 2021. China's COVID Vaccines Have Been Crucial—Now Immunity Is Waning. *Nature* 598: 398–99. [CrossRef] [PubMed]
Manning, Robert A. 2021. The U.S.-China Relationship Has Entered a New Phase. *Foreign Policy*, December 6. Available online: https://foreignpolicy.com/2021/12/06/us-china-relationship-diplomacy-after-biden-xi-summit/ (accessed on 23 January 2022).
Martin, Peter. 2021. *China's Civilian Army. The Making of Wolf Warrior Diplomacy*. Oxford: Oxford University Press.
Ngcobo, Mabutho. 2021. Mistreatment of Africans in China During COVID-19 Outbreak: When Economic Interests Superseede All Other. *Essay Series*. African Journalism and Media in the Time of COVID-19. February. Available online: https://media.africaportal.org/documents/210223-06_AP-WITS_Essay_series_Ngcobo_Final.pdf (accessed on 1 March 2022).
Nye, Joseph S. 2020. No, the Coronavirus Will Not Change the Global Order. *Foreign Policy*, April 16. Available online: https://foreignpolicy.com/2020/04/16/coronavirus-pandemic-china-united-states-power-competition/ (accessed on 25 February 2022).
O'Hanlon, Michael E. 2019. *The Senkaku Paradox. Risking Great Power War over Small Stakes*. Washington, DC: Brookings Institution Press.
Pillsbury, Michael, ed. 2020. *A Guide to the Trump Administration's China Policy Statements*. Washington, DC: Hudson Institute.
Raman, G. Venkat, and Bappaditya Murkherjee. 2021. Is COVID-Era Assertiveness in Chinese Foreign Policy Novel? *China Report* 57: 417–32. [CrossRef]
Schweller, Randall. 2006. *Unanswered Threats: Political Constraints on the Balance of Power*. Princeton: Princeton University Press.
Scissors, Derek. 2020. *Estimating the True Number of COVID-19 Cases*. Report. Washington, DC: American Enterprise Institute, April 7. Available online: https://www.aei.org/research-products/report/estimating-the-true-number-of-chinas-COVID-19-cases/?mod=article_inline (accessed on 25 January 2022).
Seaman, John, ed. 2020. *COVID-19 and Europe-China Relations. A Country-Level Analysis*. European Think-Tank Network on China (ETNC). Special Report. Paris: IFRI.
Shambaugh, David. 2020. *Where Great Powers Meet: America and China in Southeast Asia*. Oxford: Oxford University Press.

Sheehy, Thomas P., and Jospeh Asunka. 2021. Countering China on the Continent: A Look at African Views. Afrobarometer Data Reveals Africans Who Feel Positively about Chinese Influence Are More Likely to Hold Positive Views of U.S. Influence. In *Analysis and Commentaries*. Washington, DC: United States Institute of Peace. Available online: https://www.usip.org/publications/2021/06/countering-china-continent-look-african-views (accessed on 24 February 2022).

Silver, Laura, Kat Devlin, and Christine Huang. 2020. Unfavorable Views of China Reach Historic Highs in Many Countries. Majorities Say China Has Handled COVID-19 Outbreak Poorly. *Pew Research Center*, October 6. Available online: https://www.pewresearch.org/global/2020/10/06/unfavorable-views-of-china-reach-historic-highs-in-many-countries/ (accessed on 23 January 2022).

Silver, Laura. 2021. China's International Image Remains Broadly Negative as Views of the U.S. Rebound. June 30. Available online: https://www.pewresearch.org/fact-tank/2021/06/30/chinas-international-image-remains-broadly-negative-as-views-of-the-u-s-rebound/ (accessed on 25 February 2022).

Sun, Yun. 2020. China's "Wolf Warrior" Diplomacy in the COVID-19 Crisis. *The Asan Forum*, November–December. Available online: https://theasanforum.org/chinas-wolf-warrior-diplomacy-in-the-COVID-19-crisis/ (accessed on 25 February 2022).

Wang, Orange. 2021. China's Zero-COVID Strategy Risks Isolating It from Trade Partners as US Tensions Rise, Expert Says. *South China Morning Post*, February 18. Available online: https://www.scmp.com/economy/china-economy/article/3160140/chinas-zero-COVID-strategy-risks-isolating-it-trade-partners (accessed on 24 January 2022).

Xi, Jinping. 2017. Secure a Decisive Victory in Building a Moderately Prosperous Society in All Respects and Strive for the Great Success of Socialism with Chinese Characteristics for a New Era. Delivered at the 19th National Congress of the Communist Party of China. October 18. Available online: https://www.mfa.gov.cn/ce/ceil/eng/zt/19thCPCNationalCongress/W020171120127269060039.pdf (accessed on 26 February 2022).

Xinhua. 2020a. Xinhua Headlines: China Timely Shares COVID-19 Information, Advances Int'l Cooperation. *Xinhua*, April 7. Available online: http://www.xinhuanet.com/english/2020-04/07/c_138952140.htm (accessed on 28 February 2022).

Xinhua. 2020b. Fighting COVID-19: China in Action. State Council Information Office of the People's Republic of China. *Xinhua*, June 7. Available online: http://www.xinhuanet.com/english/2020-06/07/c_139120424.htm (accessed on 24 February 2022).

Xinhua. 2021a. Xi Announces Supplying Africa with Additional 1b COVID-19 Vaccine Doses, Pledges to Jointly Implement Nine Programs. In *Xinhua*; November 30. Available online: http://en.cppcc.gov.cn/2021-11/30/c_686180.htm (accessed on 25 January 2022).

Xinhua. 2021b. Full Text: China: Democracy that Works. *Xinhua*, December 4. Available online: http://www.news.cn/english/2021-12/04/c_1310351231.htm (accessed on 24 January 2022).

Yang, Mary. 2022. Southeast Asian Traders Are Paying the Cost of China's Border Policies. *Foreign Policy*, February 18. Available online: https://foreignpolicy.com/2022/02/18/asean-china-COVID-trade-border/ (accessed on 25 February 2022).

Yu, Bin. 2022. Back to the Past: The Significance of Russia and China's Joint Statement. *Pacific Forum*. February 16. Available online: https://pacforum.org/publication/pacnet-8-back-to-the-past-the-significance-of-russia-and-chinas-joint-statement (accessed on 24 February 2022).

Zhao, Suisheng, ed. 2020. *China's Global Reach. The Belt and Road Initiative (BRI) and the Asian Infrastructure Investment Bank (AIIB)*. London and New York: Routledge, vols. I and II.

Zhao, Xiaoyu. 2022. Chinese nationalism during the COVID-19 pandemic: Conciliatory and confrontational discourses. *Nations and Nationalism*, January 4. [CrossRef]

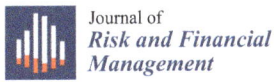

Article

To Trust or Not to Trust? COVID-19 Facemasks in China–Europe Relations: Lessons from France and the United Kingdom

Emilie Tran [1,*] and Yu-chin Tseng [2]

1 Department of Government and International Relations, Hong Kong Baptist University, Kowloon Tong, Hong Kong
2 CCKF-European Research Center on Contemporary Taiwan, University of Tübingen, 72074 Tübingen, Germany; yu-chin.tseng@uni-tuebingen.de
* Correspondence: emilietran@hkbu.edu.hk

Abstract: At the crossroads of sociology and international relations, this interdisciplinary and comparative research article explores how the COVID-19 outbreak has impacted China–Europe relations. Unfolding the critical moments of the COVID-19 outbreak, this article characterizes the evolution of China–Europe relations with regard to the facemask. This simple object of self-protection against the coronavirus strikingly became a source of contention between peoples and states. In the face of this situation, we argue that the facemask is the prism through which to illustrate (1) the transnational links between China and its overseas population, (2) the changing social perceptions of China and Chinese-looking people in European societies, and (3) the advent of China's health diplomacy and its reception in Europe. Comparing two European settings—France and the United Kingdom (UK)—the common denominator appears to be the reduced trust, if not outright distrust, between individuals and communities in the French and British contexts, and in Sino–French and Sino–British relations at the transnational level. Combining critical juncture theory and (dis)trust in international relations as our analytical framework, this article examines how the facemask became a politicized object, both between states and between Mainland China and its overseas population, as the epidemic unfolded throughout Europe. Adopting a qualitative approach, our dataset comprises the analysis of official speeches and statements; press releases; traditional and social media content (especially through hashtags such as #JeNeSuisPasUnVirus, #IAmNotAVirus, #CoronaRacism, etc.); and interviews with Chinese, French, and British community members.

Keywords: COVID-19; critical juncture; (dis)trust; health diplomacy; facemasks; racism

Citation: Tran, Emilie, and Yu-chin Tseng. 2022. To Trust or Not to Trust? COVID-19 Facemasks in China–Europe Relations: Lessons from France and the United Kingdom. *Journal of Risk and Financial Management* 15: 187. https://doi.org/10.3390/jrfm15040187

Academic Editor: Thanasis Stengos

Received: 17 January 2022
Accepted: 5 April 2022
Published: 18 April 2022

Publisher's Note: MDPI stays neutral with regard to jurisdictional claims in published maps and institutional affiliations.

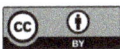

Copyright: © 2022 by the authors. Licensee MDPI, Basel, Switzerland. This article is an open access article distributed under the terms and conditions of the Creative Commons Attribution (CC BY) license (https://creativecommons.org/licenses/by/4.0/).

1. Introduction

Along with climate change, the rise of China is arguably one of the most important developments in the current century. Some claim that the China–US rivalry could be *the* defining feature of 21st century global politics, as it "may lead to escalation to cold war or even hot war" (Zhao 2022, p. 2). Therefore, scholars and policy pundits have analysed how China's rise has been transforming the world order, and the potential consequences for the other players of the international system. This article examines how China's rise has effectively affected China–Europe relations in the COVID-19 era.

Having previously contended that COVID-19 created a critical juncture in China–Europe relations, and China–France relations in particular (Tran 2022), the present article further elaborates on the processes at work in this critical juncture. Introduced by Lipset and Rokkan (1967) in their seminal work, a critical juncture is a turning point that is triggered by one kind of cause; the latter alters the state of affairs with persistent effects. In this article, we contend that China's health diplomacy campaign against COVID-19 is the straw that broke the camel's back, or the critical juncture in China–Europe relations. Since Beijing adopted its reform and opening-up policy in the late 1970s, Europe has been a key stakeholder in

China's rise in the global economy. The crackdown on the pro-democracy movement in June 1989 only momentarily shattered the China–Europe partnership. Since the second half of the 2010s, however, President Xi Jinping's multibillion infrastructure plan to connect Asia to Europe, aka the Belt and Road Initiative (BRI), has been a real test for Europe's cohesion, and has contributed to the change in attitude of the West towards China. At the 2017 inaugural Belt and Road Forum, the EU delegates startled their Chinese hosts by refusing to endorse the BRI. In September 2018, the EU issued its own response to China's plan, in the form of an alternative development project titled, "Connecting Europe and Asia—Building Blocks for an EU Strategy" (European Commission 2018). Additionally, in March 2019, the EU unveiled its document, "EU-China—A Strategic Outlook", which concomitantly calls China a partner, a competitor, and systemic rival (European Commission 2019). In Spring 2020, whereas the Europeans went into lockdown amidst their first COVID-19 outbreak, China, which had just recovered from the first wave, delivered surgical masks, protective gear, respirators, and ventilators worldwide, in addition to providing loans and medical assistance (Zhao 2020; Zoubir and Tran 2021). The Chinese Communist Party-State tried to enact a new role (Harnisch et al. 2015), showing a caring outlook, not only towards its nationals living overseas, i.e., the Chinese diaspora, but also to the world at large. In its special report titled, *COVID-19 and Europe-China Relations: A country-level analysis* (Seaman and French Institute of International Relations 2020), the consortium of the European think Tank Network on China found that the health crisis has served as "a catalyst for a number of trends that have been shaping Europe–China relations in recent years, while in other ways it has turned the tables" (Seaman and French Institute of International Relations 2020, p. 7), thus effectively ending the "age of "naiveté" towards China" (ibid, p. 10). Qi et al. (2021) argue that Beijing's medical aid revived Orientalist discourses and the fear of a Yellow Peril, in their framing analysis of China's mask diplomacy in Europe early on in the COVID-19 pandemic. As a matter of fact, in 2020–2021, Europeans across the continent expressed an exceptionally high level of unfavourable sentiment towards China (Silver et al. 2020, 2021).

Therefore, the core question that this article seeks to answer is: why did China's medical aid and health diplomacy campaign fail to win the hearts and minds of the people in Europe? We break down our core research question into three sub-questions. Firstly, what was the state of China–Europe relations prior to the pandemic? Secondly, how did the Europeans and the Chinese react during the pandemic? Thirdly, what were the consequences of the Europeans' and Chinese (re)actions?

We address the above questions by arguing that the answers lie in the question of trust. Contributing to the recently revived literature on trust in international relations, this article aims to disentangle the intricate transnational relations between China and Europe in the first half of 2020.

This article outlines the different phases of the COVID-19 critical juncture in two European countries, namely France and the United Kingdom. These countries are the focus of the article for two reasons. Firstly, among Western European powers, France and the UK have had the longest and most eventful relationship with China: from former colonial powers to strategic partners. Due to their historical relations, France and the UK are also the two European countries that have the largest community of Chinese immigrants and their descendants (Statista 2022).

Intersecting critical juncture theory with the concept of trust in the international relations literature, this article adopts a comparative approach to show how (dis)trust effectively shapes transnational relationships by analysing it in a two-level approach: at the government and community levels in France and the UK, respectively. Following the presentation of our Theoretical Framework (Section 2) and Materials and Research Methods (Section 3), the remainder of the article analyses our Findings (Section 4).

2. Theoretical Framework

2.1. Critical Juncture

Collier and Munck (2017) have defined five stages in framing a critical juncture analysis: (1) the antecedent conditions, (2) the cleavage or shock, leading to (3) the critical juncture itself, (4) the mechanisms of the production of the critical juncture's legacy, and (5) the legacy itself, in the form of durable, stable institutions. Applying Collier and Munck's stages, we contend that the critical juncture in China–Europe relations consists of the following five stages (Figure 1). First, amid the mounting distrust towards China (Section 4.1: *Antecedent Conditions*), Europe also showed solidarity with China as the latter battled against the outbreak in winter 2020, despite concerns about the origin of the SARS-Cov-2 virus (Section 4.2: *Cleavage*). When COVID-19 hit Europe, forcing it into lockdown, China politicised its medical aid and health diplomacy campaign to which France and the UK reacted in a "battle of narratives" (Section 4.3: *Critical Juncture*). At the community level, recalling a Chinese idiom "offering fuel in snowy weather (雪中送炭)", the Chinese state offered transnational support to the overseas Chinese living in the UK and France, which effectively led to the production of the critical juncture legacy (Section 4.4: *Production of the legacy*). Lastly, the *legacy* (Section 4.5) consisted of heightened discrimination and mounting distrust against Asian-looking people and China.

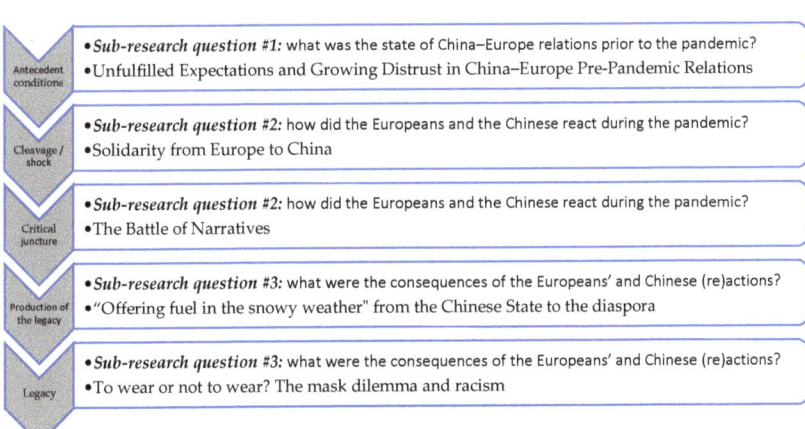

Figure 1. Critical juncture-framed research questions.

2.2. Trust

Trust (and its antonym, distrust) is identified as one of the backbones of social, economic, and political life. This concept has long been discussed in management studies focusing on trust as rational prediction and calculation or seeing it as an affect-based belief in moral character (Wicks et al. 1999). Trust in each other, in public institutions, and trust between states are all essential for the functioning of any society. Particularly during public health emergencies such as COVID-19, governments rely on public trust from their people to achieve successful COVID-19 responses (Saechang et al. 2021; Pak et al. 2021). While Cole et al. (2021), in this Special Issue, point out the role of transparency in building up trust through analysing trust in the crisis of trust, the present article looks at trust through the prism of facemask provision in two dimensions, at the international relations level (state to state), and between the state and its overseas population, against the background of COVID-19. For this purpose, the authors discuss three levels of trust.

First, trust is defined in its most basic form as an analysis of the relationship between a subject (the one who trusts) and an object (the one who is trusted). Trust has a moralistic variant, faith in a generalized other. Having trust in those who are not like 'us', rather than trusting only the familiar ones and excluding others, is what serves as the foundation of a better society (Uslaner 2002). On the contrary, a lack of trust in others can take an extreme form, such as COVID-19 related hate crimes against Asian-looking people, which will be discussed later in the article.

Second, in the field of international relations (IR), trust is an underemphasised concept that appears only occasionally in the IR scholarship (Booth and Wheeler 2010). Most often, when applied, it takes the form of an epiphenomenal by-product of cooperation among sovereign actors in the international system (Torsten 2016; Ruzicka and Wheeler 2010, pp. 69–85; Leach and Sabatier 2005, pp. 491–503; McGillivray and Smith 2000, pp. 809–24). As Axelrod (1990) pointed out, trust has seldom been considered a central variable for cooperation in the past. More recently, the concepts of trust and trust-building have re-emerged in the IR literature, for they provide an additional way not only to comprehend but also to influence international politics (Hoffman 2002, pp. 375–401). Kydd (2005) differentiates between trust and being trustworthy and concludes that strong states can promote cooperation if they are relatively trustworthy, and even if states strongly mistrust each other, they can still reassure each other and cooperate, provided that they are trustworthy. In this sense, Hoffman's idea of trust, "a willingness to take risks on the behaviour of others based on the belief that potential trustees will 'do what is right'", is more similar to trustworthiness (Hoffman 2002). Lieberthal and Wang (2012) and Chan (2017) argue that strategic distrust has underpinned the rivalry between China and the West. Since the mid-2010s, Chinese and European officials have reiterated the importance of restoring trust in their respective speeches (Tran and Zoubir 2022).

Third, this article examines trust at a level that has been overlooked, i.e., the transnational relationship between the Chinese state in the homeland and its overseas population during the pandemic. In China, the level of trust among the people in their government increased from 76% to 91% from 2016 to 2021, but underwent a significant decline in 2020 (82%), which was most likely related to the government's responses to COVID-19 (Statista 2021). The clear reduction in trust in the government reminded Beijing of the importance of trust-building among its nationals, including those abroad, who Xi described as the "magic weapons" and the public diplomats (Thunø 2018) of China's global influence making. However, the trust of the overseas population in their native country has not been sufficiently researched. Does emigration influence people's level of trust in government? How does a government maintain or enhance trust among its overseas population? This paper seeks to approach these questions by looking at the transnational mobilisation of masks between China and Europe in the context of the pandemic.

Through the case of the mobilization of help from Europe to China and the return of help in France and the UK, we examine the ways in which the regimes exercise external power transnationally through networked structures, such as embassies and associations of fellow provincials or occupations, which regulate access to the home country for the overseas population and function as "an extension and in the service of the authoritarian state at home"(Brand 2008, p. 111).

Consulting these ideas of trust, we inquire about the nature of trust and the aggravated mistrust in China–Europe relations and examine how this brought the China–Europe relations to a critical juncture. Figure 2 in the Conclusion summarises our findings on how trust plays out in a multilevel approach to China–Europe relations.

3. Materials and Research Methods

This article is based on qualitative research carried out through desktop data collection. Qualitative data offer a rich portrayal and explanation of this study's subjects, especially the evolution of inter-state and infra-state relationships, providing first-hand insights into the transnational mobilisation of medical aid between China and Europe, and the lived experiences of people. The materials for our study consist of:

(i) Chinese and European governmental statements, press conferences, and announcements from 2018 to April 2020.

(ii) Chinese, French, and British media reports and web contents from January to April 2020, including but not limited to *The Global Times*, Xinhua, *Le Monde*, *Le Figaro*, *The Guardian*, CGTN, France Television, LCI, and the BBC.
(iii) Posts on social media and discussion forums from December 2019 to May 2020.
(iv) A total of 21 in-depth interviews with overseas Chinese in Europe, conducted in March–April–May 2020.

Applying a frame analysis to materials (i) and (ii)[1], we studied the language used by government officials and journalists in China, France, and the UK to refer to the other party, from the first COVID-19 outbreak in winter 2020 to the end of April 2020 as China deployed its high-profile mask diplomacy. A constructivist method devised by Erving Goffman (1974), frame analysis is particularly appropriate in our study to understand a given situation (the pandemic) and activities (China's health diplomacy campaign and the ensuing battle of narratives between China and Europe).

In addition, using digital ethnography techniques, we followed campaigners on Twitter[2] and WeChat. The latter is the most popular social media among the Chinese. We observed chat groups' discussion forums as well as the official WeChat pages of Chinese associations, such as the local branches of the Overseas Chinese Federation and the Chinese Students and Scholars Association. Digital ethnography is an online research method used to study the communities created through ICT-based social interactions: "communication and situations mediated through digital platforms become a significant part of what actors do, of their interactions and practices, the ethnographer needs to have part in them" (Hine 2015, pp. 8–9). The collection of digital ethnographic data allowed us to delve into the activities, actions and reactions of the Chinese living in France in winter and spring 2020.

Last but not least, we conducted interviews by phone and videoconference calls. Recruited via snowball samplings, the respondents were students from Mainland China, Hong Kong, and Taiwan in academic mobility in Europe at the time of the interview. In a safe and comfortable environment, the respondents provided an actor-based elaboration of the situations experienced. All 21 respondents offered valuable insights that led to a deeper understanding of transnational solidarity, discrimination, and identity struggle.

4. Findings

4.1. Antecedent Conditions: Unfulfilled Expectations and Growing Distrust in China–Europe Pre-Pandemic Relations

The assumption of Western governments had long been that, as China grew economically and became more intertwined with global trade, it would transform inexorably into a liberal democracy. This Hegelian outlook, popularized by Francis Fukuyama's book, *The End of History* (Fukuyama 1992), assumed that the world moved inevitably towards democracy and free-market economics. Yet, after the so-called 'lost-decade' under President Hu Jintao and Premier Wen Jiabao, his successor Xi Jinping has led China authoritatively and unfolded the 'Third Revolution' (Economy 2018), in stark contrast to Deng Xiaoping's 'Second Revolution' of the 1970s–1980s, which was characterized by greater political and economic opening, and a low-profile foreign policy [韜光養晦, 有所作為] or [韜光养晦]. Having pursued the reform of state-owned enterprises, improved the country's innovation capacity, and enhanced air quality, China has become an economic powerhouse and a global trade partner. However, its domestic market remains limited to foreign companies, and illegal intellectual appropriation and forced technology transfers have not ended. Socially, the State imposes social control and limits public criticism from civil rights lawyers, independent journalists, and ethnic and religious minorities (Human Rights Watch 2020). On top of that, there are contending issues regarding the South China Sea, industrial and scientific espionage (Hvistendahl 2020), and influential politics in Western democracies that erode trust in China in many ways (Hamilton 2018; Diamond and Schell 2019; Lulu 2019). Thus, not surprisingly, the evolution of China has not followed the trajectory that Westerners had anticipated, despite Western pressures, especially since 9/11 (Börzel 2015; Carothers and Ottaway 2010).

Against this background, the West's distrust in China has grown considerably in different places in the world (Tran and Zoubir 2022). Unquestionably, COVID-19 exacerbated the US–China rivalry (Wang 2019). Indeed, the United States emphasized that China challenges "American power, influence, and interests, attempting to erode American security and prosperity" (The White House 2017) by "contesting [US] geopolitical advantages and trying to change the international order in [its] favor" and by "investing billions of dollars in infrastructure across the globe", which will "reinforce its geopolitical aspirations" (The White House 2017). If in the Middle East and Africa China's economic policies and infrastructure diplomacy are seen as South–South development cooperation, the West perceives them as Beijing's geopolitical gains, confirming its strategic mistrust towards China.

Although Chinese and European senior leaders meet regularly and maintain steady government-to-government dialogue, the EU has grown wary of Beijing's global influence. China's multi-billion infrastructure plans, the Belt and Road Initiative (BRI), and other foreign policy programmes have generated distrust regarding China's actual intentions. This distrust has become a major impediment to the BRI and a challenge to Europe's unity, as well as a strain on Europe's relations with China. Consequently, EU delegates refused to endorse, as a bloc, China's BRI (European Parliament 2018; Phillips 2017). In 2018, the EU issued its own response (adopted in 2019) to China's BRI in the form of an alternative development project (European Commission 2018). In 2019, the EU unveiled a new and unequivocal criticism of Beijing, depicting China as "an economic competitor in the pursuit of technological leadership, and a systemic rival promoting alternative models of governance" (European Commission 2019). This marked a sharp change in the Sino–European relationship, a view which was not limited to the policymakers but also extended to EU citizens. Surveys demonstrated that most Europeans held a negative view of China (European Commission 2016).

In March 2019, European leaders reiterated that "Europe must be united and have a coherent message" towards China (France24 2019), to which President Xi responded by first acknowledging the trust deficit in global affairs, before adding that "We cannot let mutual suspicion get the better of us", calling all parties to cooperatively lay the foundations of mutual trust (France24 2019). On 23 July 2020, US Secretary of State Michael Pompeo emphasized that the new US policy towards China would rest on "distrust" (US Department of State 2020).

Against this backdrop of mounting tensions between China and the West, this article argues that the COVID-19 pandemic has created a critical juncture in China–Europe relations, where the trust deficit has translated into outright distrust.

4.2. Cleavage: Solidarity from Europe to China

Our research has uncovered that China has enacted two seemingly opposite roles: on the one hand, it appears to be a suspicious international actor, accused of covering up information with regard to the origin of the outbreak and the actual figures of COVID-19 cases; on the other hand, it promotes itself as a benevolent global health actor, providing aid where needed, and supporting its aid with a forceful and at times aggressive global communication campaign. These two roles of China created wariness, distrust, and condemnation among certain European recipient countries of China's health diplomacy, especially in the UK and France. In this section, we examine the critical juncture in China–Europe relations, focusing on the cases of France and the UK, to exhibit the ways in which the relations with China evolved over the pandemic and China's pursuit of a new role.

In the first quarter of 2020, when China was struggling with the new coronavirus, Europe and other countries worldwide stepped in to show solidarity with China by providing medical provisions and personal protective equipment. We observe that the solidarity from Europe came at both the state level and meso level organized by individuals or associations.

At the state level, following the outbreak in Wuhan, China received massive donations of masks and medical equipment from a dozen international organizations and many countries, including not so wealthy and developing countries (Zoubir and Tran 2021), and the US, amid the Sino–US trade war (Zhao 2020). The objective was to help China contain the coronavirus. The EU alone donated more than 50 tons of equipment in January 2020, as the President of the European Commission, Ursula von der Leyen, recalled (European Commission 2020). Having reached out to his Chinese counterpart through two phone calls (20 January and 18 February), President Macron ordered the delivery of 17 tons of medical supplies (protective suits, gloves, hydro-alcoholic gels and 560,000 face masks) from France's strategic stocks. In an event organized by the Chinese ambassador to the UK, Liu Xiaoming, the Chinese residing in the UK shipped almost GBP 400,000 worth of medical supplies to the doctors fighting coronavirus in Wuhan on 1 February 2020 (Jia 2020). The European Think Tank Network on China issued a report that detailed the actual assistance sent by European states, country by country, to China (Seaman and French Institute of International Relations 2020).

Our digital ethnographic observations show that solidarity support at the non-state level, such as from the UK to China, by regional associations of fellow provincials (同鄉会 tong xiang hui), business associations (商会 shang hui), and student associations, was mainly organized between January and February 2020. These associations represent the three main groups of Chinese people living in the UK. Solidarity with China was shown mainly through shipping much needed medical supplies to the country. At the community level, many *tong xiang hui* and business associations, such as the UK Henan Chinese Association, the UK Tianjin Business Association, and the London Chinatown Chinese Association (Tianjin Federation of Returned Overseas Chinese 2020; Sohu 2020; Oushinet 2020), just to name a few, organized donations to help regions they had ties within China. The Chinese Students and Scholars Association (CSSA-UK), as well as donations to hospitals in China, provided cultural solidarity by organizing Chinese students studying in the UK to compose and produce a music video to show solidarity with Wuhan. The CCSA-UK was established in 1988 and is supervised by the Education Section of the Embassy of the People's Republic of China in the United Kingdom. It is one of the largest Chinese associations in the UK with around 220,000 members. It showed strong organizational capacity and also played a crucial role in organizing the solidarity activities at a later stage.

The Chinese authorities acknowledged this show of solidarity from the international community. On 1 February 2020, CGTN ran a headline: "China thanks EU donations to assist relief efforts during coronavirus outbreak". (CGTN 2020a; Xinhua 2020b). On 20 March 2020, one could read "Xinhua Headlines: China returns solidarity with Europe in COVID-19 battle" (Xinhua 2020c), which emphasized the fact that Europe had made the first gesture of solidarity.

4.3. Critical Juncture: The Battle of Narratives

As COVID-19 cases were brought under control in China, Beijing immediately started to "fight back" against the repeated accusations from foreign countries, and those in the West in particular, of having covered up information regarding the virus since late 2019. Against this background, in February 2020, in a meeting of the Politburo Standing Committee, Xi indicated the importance of telling a good anti-epidemic story of China to display the solidarity of the Chinese people domestically and internationally (The State Council of the People's Republic of China 2020b). In March, it was emphasised by Wang Yi, the Vice Foreign Minister, that his diplomatic work would actively take part in anti-pandemic diplomacy to gain international support, to promote international collaborations, to safeguard Chinese citizens' rights abroad, and to vigorously engage in propaganda to *tell good anti-pandemic stories* (好中国抗疫故事 jiang hao zhongguo kangyi gushi) (The State Council of the People's Republic of China 2020a). Thus, as the pandemic started to seriously hit Europe, where some countries had some of the largest numbers of coronavirus cases in the world in March 2020 and struggled to contain the spread of the virus, Beijing seized the chance to emerge as a partner that was eager to provide much needed aid. China provided help to European countries as an experienced fighter against the virus and a benevolent international friend, repeatedly using the term "offering fuel in the snowy weather".

Health diplomacy has been part of Chinese diplomacy since the early days of the People's Republic of China, and all the more so in the 21st century. Therefore, it is not surprising that the Chinese Party-State sought to promote it at a time when many countries were struggling to respond to the COVID-19 pandemic. This time, China also activated its BRI networks to carry out its mask diplomacy to supply aid and act as a "responsible great power" (Rudolf and Stiftung Wissenschaft Und Politik 2021). What started as a massive health crisis actually turned into a political opportunity for China: at last, Beijing could take on a role traditionally played by the great Western powers. Moreover, mask diplomacy served a dual role: to sweep its failure in not containing the virus at the early stages of the outbreak under the carpet, and to gain domestic public support (Kowalski 2021).

However, in order to presume the role of a global health promoter, China needed a new narrative to combat the prevailing distrust in the international community, mainly the doubts over the reporting and origins of COVID-19, and to enhance trust among overseas Chinese, who are "magic weapons" (法宝 fabao) of Beijing's influence diplomacy, according to Xi (Brady 2017).

As China had presumably won its battle, even though the exact figures of infected and deceased patients were and continue to be questionable, China was ahead of other countries in terms of medical staff experience, having treated more than 80,000 patients with COVID-19. China also considerably increased its production capacity of protective equipment (including face masks) and ventilators, much needed items that other countries had already been relying on Chinese companies to provide. On 26 March 2020, *The Global Times* published an infographic presenting the various initiatives of Chinese health diplomacy in the fight against the COVID-19 pandemic (Global Times 2020). By providing its assistance, particularly technical, China sought to convince its partners of its exemplary nature, and to make people forget its errors and responsibilities in the initial management of the crisis. Indeed, Beijing, having apparently been aware of the risk of human-to-human transmission from the end of December 2019, failed to notify the WHO in due course, whereas Taiwan had been trying to alert the WHO about that risk, even though China has forbidden it from joining the WHO. This likely aggravated the pre-existing distrust based on China's past mishandling of outbreak reporting and lack of transparency and cooperation.

China's attempt to change the narrative can be seen in a column published on 24 March 2020, in *The People's Daily* which, in addition to urging all countries to join the Health Silk Road, stated that "China has, in an open and transparent manner, and responsible, informed all parties of the epidemic in a timely manner and worked closely with WHO and affected countries" (People's Daily 2020). China tried to convince developing countries, but also many European countries, that it, alone, was a trustworthy partner able to help them in this unprecedented health crisis and that its system of governance was the one that was most able to cope with it. Within the broader framework of the Sino–American competition, its objectives were to present itself with a better posture than the United States, while discrediting the Western democracies (Ambassade de Chine en France 2020):

> Since the Republic of Korea, Japan and Singapore, which are Asian democracies, are succeeding in controlling the epidemic, why are old democracies like Europe and the United States not succeeding?
>
> [. . .]
>
> Asian countries, including China, have been particularly successful in their fight against COVID-19 because they have that sense of community and civility that Western democracies lack. (Ambassade de Chine en France 2020)

This attempt escalated online. A case in point is the unprecedented offensive by the PRC's embassy in France that actively promoted Beijing's narrative on social media, on its website, and in French media. As illustrated by our research projects, "Chinese Twitter" (in 2020) and "China's Twitter Diplomacy: Content and Impact" (in 2021–2022) (Thunø 2021, 2022), the Chinese embassy and, to a lesser extent, the Consulate of China in Strasbourg and the Consulate of China in Lyon became very active on Twitter in August 2019, and February and March 2020, respectively. Although the Chinese embassy in Paris created its Twitter account in August 2019 when the new ambassador, Lu Shaye, took office, it suddenly became active on 4 February 2020, retweeting the WHO Director-General Tedros Adhanom Ghebreyesus. It subsequently tweeted several times a day, mostly about COVID-19-related issues. Then, the tweets began to spread rumours and conspiracy theories, which were not conducive to trust, suggesting that COVID-19 had originated in the United States and was brought to China by the US military—a story supported by other Chinese officials. In March–April 2020, the embassy also published several anonymous editorial-style articles on its website, which aimed at "restoring the distorted facts" presented by Western media, politicians and experts" who intended to slander China. Titled «Rétablir des faits distordus—Observations d'un diplomate chinois en poste à Paris» [Restoring distorted facts—Observations of a Chinese diplomat stationed in Paris], the articles mixed real facts with false or unfounded allegations, denigrated Western democracies' handling of the crisis, and advanced the official narrative of the PRC's success. The most aggressive article, for example, published on 12 April, promoted the theory that the virus could have originated in the United States, accused French members of Parliament of supporting a declaration by Taiwan that called Tedros a "nigger", and blamed the personnel of retirement homes for "having abandoned their positions overnight, collectively deserting and leaving their inhabitants to die of hunger and disease." The French Minister of Foreign Affairs, Jean-Yves Le Drian, summoned Lu Shaye on April 14 to express his disapproval of the embassy's criticisms towards the Western response to the coronavirus pandemic (Le Monde 2020). The Chinese embassy tried to explain the situation as a misunderstanding, blaming the media for having distorted its intended meaning (Ambassade de la République Populaire de Chine en République Française 2020). Nonetheless, on 24 May, the embassy's Twitter account published a cartoon with the comment "Qui est le prochain?" [Who's next?]. The polemical drawing accused the United States of being responsible for the conflicts in Iraq, Libya, Syria, Ukraine, Venezuela and, ultimately, Hong Kong. Although the embassy claimed that its Twitter account had been hacked and deleted the controversial post, netizens doubted the embassy's word (LCI 2020). Lu also made multiple appearances in the French media to defend the Chinese narrative. The Chinese embassy in France reflected Beijing's then diplomatic approach to public diplomacy, one that is more proactive and aggressive, and dubbed "Wolf Warrior" diplomacy after the Chinese blockbuster movie *Wolf Warrior 2*, released in 2018. This new approach has been observed in many countries since then, especially in Europe.

Anglo–Chinese relations, or to be more precise, UK–China business relations, have been hit severely by COVID-19 as well as the online battle of narratives. Some even predict that the pandemic will spell the end of what a former British finance minister called the "golden era", since 2013, when Huawei confirmed a 1.3 billion investment in the UK and the Prime Minister David Cameron promised that the UK and China would have a long-term relationship during his visit to China. Furthermore, the UK was the first major Western country to join the China-led Asian Infrastructure Investment Bank (AIIB). In October 2015, Xi paid a State Visit to the UK shortly after the Chancellor of the Exchequer, George Osborne, spoke of "a golden era" for the UK–China relationship in September. The Golden Era was mentioned again to mark the visit of the Prime Minister Theresa May to China in early 2018. Yet, when the Hong Kong issue started to become salient in 2019, the UK politicians started to show dissent towards China; eventually, the government openly expressed its concern about the imposing of the national security law in HK and set out plans for British national (overseas) status holders. Meanwhile, in July 2020, the UK Government committed to the removal of Huawei equipment from the UK's 5G network by 2027.

In response to the rapid souring of the UK–China relationship from a trusted business partner to a distrusted opponent, China's narrative has also become more and more aggressive. This can be observed from a series of statements made by China's ambassador Liu Xiaoming (Seaman and French Institute of International Relations 2020). He is one of the

Wolf Warriors, a prominent defender of China on social media with over 100,000 followers on Twitter. He once fully denied any abuse of Uighurs in Xinjiang in a BBC interview and firmly defended China's imposition of the National Security Law in Hong Kong. With the UK's opening to the Hong Kong British National (Overseas) visa, the UK–China relationship continues to ebb, and China's aggressive stance will also be continued by Liu's successor, Zheng Zuguang, who has already been banned from entering Parliament.

4.4. Production of the Legacy: "Offering Fuel in the Snowy Weather" from the Chinese State to the Diaspora

On a par with the solidarity shown by the UK to China in early 2020, the "help" from China to the UK was also twofold, at the government level and the local level, and they were usually inseparable from each other (LCI 2020). At the local level, the help from China mainly came from Chinese people living in the UK and UK business partners. In terms of Chinese people living in the UK, there are long-term migrants, overseas Chinese who have lived abroad for a longer period and established a life abroad, and temporary migrants who currently live in the UK. The latter might become long-term migrants in the future, but to date they live only temporarily in the UK; they usually came to the UK with a clear purpose, such as to work or study.

At the state level, on 28 March 2020, the Joint Working Group from the Shandong province arrived in the UK. This trip brought to the UK not only medical supplies but also doctors and Shandong local government officials, including the Deputy Director of the Standing Committee of the People's Congress of Shandong and the Secretary of the Provincial Party Committee (Xinhua 2020a). It was indicated that the purpose of this visit was to assist Chinese citizens in the UK, following Xi's instruction to strengthen China's care for overseas Chinese citizens in the Politburo meeting. Xi also had a telephone conversation with the Prime Minister Boris Johnson in late March to emphasize the importance of protecting the health and safety of Chinese citizens overseas, and expressed his hope that Britain would take measures in safeguarding the health, safety, and legitimate rights of Chinese nationals, in particular those studying in the UK (CGTN 2020b). From late March to May 2020, the Federation of Returned Overseas Chinese (侨联 qiaolian) and overseas friendship associations (海外联谊会 haiwai lianyihui) in China, especially the ones in the emigration regions, released news about how many medical supplies they had organized to send to Chinese citizens living abroad in return for the favour they had received earlier. It was constantly emphasized that the natal China always cared about the safety and wellbeing of the overseas Chinese (China United Front News Network 2020). Apart from allocating medical supplies to Chinese students in cooperation with local associations of fellow provincials, the Chinese Students and Scholars Association in the United Kingdom (CSSA-UK) provided mental health support to students by organizing over three hundred mutual aid groups to include over 100,000 students. Furthermore, in corporation with medical schools in Shandong, the CSSA-UK also organized an Advising Plan (抗疫輔導計畫 kangyi fudao jihua) to match students in need with experts in Shandong for online mental health consulting and medical inquiry services (Chinese Students and Scholars Association UK 2020). This was much needed support that students usually had difficulty accessing after the lockdown. They named this series of solidarity actions "hand in hand, heart connected to heart" (手牵手, 心连心 shou qian shou xin lian xin). Later, providing medical inquiry and consulting services through WeChat groups became a common practice of other provincial associations as well. These solidarity events built trust between the state and its overseas population.

Based on the observations mentioned from our fieldwork, we argue that "health" is at the heart of both China's diplomacy and the solidarity mobilization of the Chinese overseas community in the UK. Moreover, the aim is to convey the message of a "caring homeland", and at the international level to foster international solidarity as well as trust.

4.5. Legacy: To Wear or Not to Wear? The Mask Dilemma and Racism

The last aspect of our analysis on facemasks is the undesirable impacts of mask-wearing in the French and UK societies. In France, and particularly in Paris, which concentrates the Chinese diaspora, we have shown in our previous work that the overseas Chinese had already endured discrimination for many years (Chuang et al. 2021; Tran and Chuang 2019). Therefore, when they started, as early as in December 2019, to buy face masks and gloves in pharmacies in order to ship them back to mainland China, either to friends and families back home or through e-commerce channels, this only added to their stigma. By January 2020, several pharmacies in neighbourhoods where overseas Chinese lived reported to Asian-looking clients that they had run out of stock, saying that they were out of stock due to frantic buying in December by Asians (Interviews with local pharmacies 2020). The Chinese in France continued to source and purchase protective gear and ship it to the mainland in January and February.

However, starting in February 2020, the Chinese in France, fearing the imminent arrival of the epidemic in Europe, started to source protective gear for their own use on the Internet. As they started to wear facemasks, they also became prone to hardened stigmatizing speeches and racist attacks. They had to face the dilemma between health safety and discrimination (Interview with ethnic Chinese 2020). Indeed, as the first cases of COVID-19 appeared in metropolitan France on 24 January, people of Asian origin started to be stigmatized in public places and became the victims of disrespectful behaviour and even racist insults. They were associated with the virus, as if the simple fact of having an Asian face meant being a carrier of COVID-19. On 26 January 2020, the front page of the daily newspaper, *Courrier Picard*, read "Yellow Alert" [*Alerte Jaune*]. The ensuing article was entitled "New yellow peril" [Le nouveau péril jaune], reviving a racist metaphor of the 19th century. Although the daily paper published a letter of apology justifying its editorial choices, eventually the editor had to apologize personally, and the article was eventually withdrawn from the newspaper's website. Nonetheless, the damage had been done as the clumsy and tendentious wording of certain media, along with the comments of Internet users on social media, had created a climate of psychosis in France, which led to amalgamations against the community of Chinese origin, and more generally speaking to people of Asian origin, regardless of their actual nationality. The hashtag #JeNeSuisPasUnVirus was born in response to this phenomenon and quickly relayed on social media. Faced with the recurrence of discriminatory incidents, the Chinese started to share their personal ordeals on social media and dedicated channels. Clients boycotted Chinese restaurants and businesses. However, an even larger number of these incidents took place within school premises: children and youths were stigmatized or harassed due to their origins. Chinese associations, and in particular the Association des Jeunes Chinois de France [Association of the Young Chinese in France] (Association des Jeunes Chinois de France 2020), created in 2009, were instrumental in collecting those reports and liaising with the French authorities and the civil sector to find solutions.

Meanwhile, while donations and medical supplies were being arranged at the community level to support the fight against the virus in China, Chinese people in the UK were facing hostile situations in their everyday life (Murphy 2020). As the UK has the largest number of Chinese students in Europe (120,385 engaged in higher education and 15,000 under 17 years old), it also reported many COVID-19 related incidents of hate crime against Chinese people in the UK. They were well-documented in the run up to and during the lockdown period. The assaults reported in the media, and in our own interviews, included stone throwing, individuals being spat on and assaulted, coronavirus related derogatory words being shouted, and even individuals being refused entry onto the bus due to their mask wearing. The Home Office minister told the Commons committee that Anti-Asian hate crimes went up 21% during the coronavirus crisis (Grierson 2020). At least 267 offences against Chinese people were recorded in the first three months of 2020, which was nearly three times that of the previous two years (Mercer 2020). This increased Anti-Asian hate crime was aimed at individuals, but it only shows the growing distrust towards China and anyone seemingly from and related to China. The provision of masks embodied solidarity with China on the one hand, and mask-wearing, on the other hand, marked and spurred distrust against China with regard to coronavirus.

5. Conclusions

The Introduction set out our core research question (*Why did China's medical aid and health diplomacy campaign failed to win the hearts and minds of the peoples in Europe?*) and the three sub-questions, as follows: (1) What was the state of China–Europe relations prior to the pandemic? (2) How did the Europeans and the Chinese react during the pandemic? (3) What were the consequences of the (re)actions of the Europeans and Chinese? Applying the framework of a critical juncture, this article identifies the antecedent conditions of Sino–French and Sino–British relations, the cleavage created by the outbreak of COVID-19, the battle of narratives as a critical juncture, the legacies of Beijing's mobilization of overseas Chinese in Europe, and the rampant racism targeting Asian-looking mask-wearers in Europe.

This article has shown that Sino–French and Sino–British relations prior to the pandemic had been going through a state of affairs comprising enduring concerns and issues but were certainly not confrontational or aggressive. In Spring 2020, the rift in China–Europe relations was largely widened against the background of COVID-19. China–Europe relations were then centred around a simple yet life-saving object, the medical facemask, which became a point of attention and contention, crystalizing transnational (dis)trust at the government and individual levels. Through conducting interviews, digital ethnography, and media analysis, the authors conclude that the critical juncture in China–Europe relations can be attributed to not only China's promotion of its medical aid and health diplomacy campaign, but also its engagement of aggressive Twitter diplomacy. Solidarity with China during its difficult time and the help returned by China with its experiences and resources—the mutual "offering of fuel in the snowy weather"—could have deepened their mutual trust. However, the extremely assertive discourse by their most vocal diplomats made the Chinese authorities become unpopular in both France and the UK and lose their edge and credibility, not to mention the doubts over the quality of Chinese-made medical equipment in many countries (BBC News 2020). Eventually, Beijing's diplomatic offensive in Spring 2020 proved counterproductive at the intra-state level. While distrust grew at the state level, the Chinese in Europe faced extensive racist ordeals. The distrust in China took the form of attacks on ethnic Asians wearing facemasks. Last but not least, the authors observed in the fieldwork that Beijing's campaign of telling good anti-pandemic stories of solidarity and mobilization to "offer fuel in snowy weather" to "return the help" to Europe have strengthened the transnational ties between the state and its overseas population in France and the UK.

To sum up, this article has contributed to showing that the pandemic provided China with the opportunity to stage a global political campaign, defining new forms of public diplomacy. This article's findings are threefold: (1) at the individual level, hostility towards the ethnic Asians from the host French and British societies was witnessed; (2) at the state-to-state level, China's aggressive Twitter diplomacy and the flawed health diplomacy increased the lingering distrust in China–France and China–UK relations; and, (3) the mobilization of medical aid strengthened the engagement and connection between China and the overseas Chinese in these two countries. These findings echo the three levels of trust discussed in Section 2.2, and, based on the findings, the authors have identified three levels of (dis)trust in China–Europe relations, as shown in Figure 2.

Drawing from this article's findings, the authors are now inquiring further into China's adoption of digital diplomacy, including Twitter diplomacy, as the world is recovering from the pandemic amidst a climate of enhanced tension and the war in Ukraine. More than ever, trust amongst state leaders and nations is the most important factor in regard to dialogue and peace.

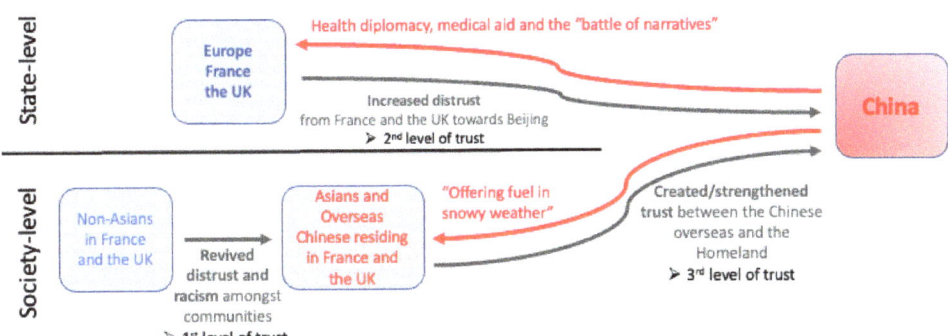

Figure 2. Multilevel (dis)trust in China–Europe relations in the early COVID-19 pandemic.

Author Contributions: Conceptualization, E.T.; methodology, E.T. and Y.-c.T.; formal analysis, E.T. and Y.-c.T.; investigation, E.T. and Y.-c.T.; resources, E.T. and Y.-c.T.; data curation, E.T. (for case study on France) and Y.-c.T. (for case study in the UK); writing—original draft preparation, E.T. and Y.-c.T.; writing—review and editing, E.T. and Y.-c.T.; visualization, E.T.; funding acquisition, E.T. All authors have read and agreed to the published version of the manuscript.

Funding: PROCORE—France/Hong Kong Joint Research Scheme, *Transnational and Transdisciplinary Lessons from the COVID-19 Pandemic*, PROCORE—France/Hong Kong Joint Research Scheme, (F-HKBU205/20), 2021–2022.

Informed Consent Statement: Informed consent was obtained from all subjects involved in the study.

Data Availability Statement: Not applicable.

Conflicts of Interest: The authors declare no conflict of interest.

Notes

1. The frame analysis of British and French media was made possible thanks to the research project titled *China's Twitter Diplomacy: Content and Impact*, funded by Aarhus University Research Foundation—AUFF NOVA, and led by Dr Mette Thunø and in which the two authors are Co-Investigators.
2. The Twitter data and analysis derive from the above research project.

References

Ambassade de Chine en France (@AmbassadeChine). 2020. Twitter. March 27, 6:04 P.M. Available online: https://twitter.com/AmbassadeChine/status/1243584778319933440?ref_src=twsrc%5Etfw%7Ctwcamp%5Etweetembed%7Ctwterm%5E1243584778319933440%7Ctwgr%5E%7Ctwcon%5Es1_&ref_url=https%3A%2F%2Fwww.leparisien.fr%2Fpolitique%2Fl-ambassadeur-de-chine-a-paris-convoque-pour-ses-propos-sur-le-coronavirus-14-04-2020-8299737.php (accessed on 30 November 2020).

Ambassade de la République Populaire de Chine en République Française. 2020. Déclaration du Porte-parole de l'Ambassade de Chine en France sur certains propos d'un article publié par l'Ambassade qui ont été déformés par la presse [Statement by the Spokesperson of the Chinese Embassy in France on Certain Remarks of an Article Published by the Embassy Which Were Distorted by the Press]. Available online: http://www.amb-chine.fr/fra/zfzj/t1772378.htm (accessed on 30 November 2020).

Association des Jeunes Chinois de France. 2020. La crise du COVID-19 en France: Position et Actions de l'AJCF. Available online: https://www.lajcf.fr/la-crise-du-COVID-19-en-france-position-et-actions-de-lajcf/ (accessed on 30 November 2020).

Axelrod, Robert. 1990. *The Evolution of Cooperation*. London: Penguin Books.

BBC News. 2020. Coronavirus: Countries Reject Chinese-Made Equipment. March 30. Available online: https://www.bbc.com/news/world-europe-52092395 (accessed on 30 November 2020).

Booth, Ken, and Nicholas Wheeler. 2010. *The Security Dilemma: Fear, Cooperation and Trust in World Politic*. Houndmills: Palgrave Macmillan.

Börzel, Tanja A. 2015. The noble west and the dirty rest? Western democracy promoters and illiberal regional powers. *Democratization* 22: 519–35. [CrossRef]

Brady, Anne-Marie. 2017. *Magic Weapons: China's Political Influence Activities under Xi Jinping*. Washington: Wilson Center, September. Available online: https://www.wilsoncenter.org/article/magic-weapons-chinas-political-influence-activities-under-xi-jinping (accessed on 30 November 2020).

Brand, Laurie. 2008. *Citizens Abroad: Emigration and the State in the Middle East and North Africa*. Edited by Paperback. Cambridge: Cambridge Univ. Press.

Carothers, Thomas, and Marina Ottaway. 2010. *Uncharted Journey: Promoting Democracy in the Middle East*. Washington, DC: Brookings Institution.
CGTN. 2020a. China Thanks EU Donations to Assist Relief Efforts during Coronavirus Outbreak. February 1. Available online: https://news.cgtn.com/news/2020-02-01/China-s-Li-EU-s-von-der-Leyen-discuss-coronavirus-outbreak-over-phone-NJg1gNIx7q/index.html (accessed on 30 November 2020).
CGTN. 2020b. Chinese President Xi Jinping Holds Phone Talks with World Leaders over COVID-19. March 24. Available online: https://news.cgtn.com/news/2020-03-24/Xi-Only-by-working-together-can-mankind-win-battle-against-COVID-19-P70OtcZl4Y/index.html (accessed on 30 November 2020).
Chan, Steve. 2017. *Trust and Distrust in Sino-American Relations: Challenge and Opportunity*. Amherst: Cambria Press.
China United Front News Network. 2020. Guonei sheqiao jigou fenfen xiang haiwai juan zhang fangyi wuzi [Domestic Overseas Chinese Institutions Have Donated Materials for Epidemic Prevention to Overseas]. Available online: http://tyzx.people.cn/BIG5/n1/2020/0415/c431923-31673976.html (accessed on 30 November 2020).
Chinese Students and Scholars Association UK. 2020. Shouqianshou xinlianxin—Shandong zhuanjia zhuli liuying xuezi beibuqu he beiaiqu kangyi jishi. [Hand in Hand, Heart to Heart—Shandong Experts Help Chinese Students Studying in the UK to Fight the Epidemic in Northern England and Northern IRELAND], July 31. Available online: https://mp.weixin.qq.com/s/w-MGs4F6zmc18rX4hBtWsQ (accessed on 30 November 2020).
Chuang, Ya-Han, Émilie Tran, and Hélène le Bail. 2021. From Silence to Action: The Chinese in France. *Global Dialogue. Magazine of the International Sociological Association* 11. Available online: https://globaldialogue.isa-sociology.org/articles/from-silence-to-action-the-chinese-in-france (accessed on 1 January 2022).
Cole, Alister, Julien S. Baker, and Dionysios Stivas. 2021. Trust, Transparency and Transnational Lessons from COVID-19. *Journal of Risk and Financial Management* 14: 607. [CrossRef]
Collier, David, and Gerardo L. Munck. 2017. Building Blocks and Methodological Challenges: A Framework for Studying Critical Junctures. *Qualitative and Multi-Method Research* 15: 2–9.
Diamond, Larry, and Orville Schell. 2019. *China's Influence and American Interest: Promoting Constructive Vigilance*. Stanford: Hoover Institution Press Publication.
Economy, Elizabeth. 2018. *Xi Jinping and the New Chinese State*. Oxford: Oxford University Press.
European Commission. 2016. Future of Europe. In *Special Eurobarometer 451*. Available online: https://data.europa.eu/euodp/en/data/dataset/S2131_86_1_451_ENG (accessed on 23 July 2020).
European Commission. 2018. Joint Communication to the European Parliament, The Council, The European Economic and Social Committee, The Committee of the Regions and the European Investment Bank. Connecting Europe and Asia—Building blocks for an EU Strategy. Available online: https://www.eeas.europa.eu/sites/default/files/joint_communication_-_connecting_europe_and_asia_-_building_blocks_for_an_eu_strategy_2018-09-19.pdf (accessed on 1 January 2022).
European Commission. 2019. EU-China-A Strategic Outlook. Available online: https://ec.europa.eu/commission/sites/beta-political/files/communication-eu-china-a-strategic-outlook.pdf (accessed on 23 July 2020).
European Commission. 2020. President Ursula Von der Leyen on Her Phone Call with the Prime Minister of China LI Keqiang. Available online: https://audiovisual.ec.europa.eu/en/topnews/M-004589 (accessed on 30 November 2020).
European Parliament, Directorate-General for Internal Policies. 2018. The New Silk Route—Opportunities and Challenges for EU Transport. p. 15. Available online: https://www.europarl.europa.eu/RegData/etudes/STUD/2018/585907/IPOL_STU(2018)585907_EN.pdf (accessed on 30 November 2020).
France24. 2019. Discours d'Emmanuel Macron, Xi Jinping, Angela Merkel et Jean-Claude Juncker à l'Elysée. Available online: https://www.youtube.com/watch?v=FWd55m2n_0g (accessed on 30 November 2020).
Fukuyama, Francis. 1992. *The End of History and the Last Man*. New York: Free Press.
Global Times. 2020. Available online: https://twitter.com/globaltimesnews/status/1243074378704678918 (accessed on 30 November 2020).
Goffman, Erving. 1974. *Frame Analysis: An Essay on the Organization of Experience*. New York: Harper Torchbooks.
Grierson, Jamie. 2020. Anti-Asian Hate Crimes up 21% in UK during Coronavirus Crisis. *The Guardian*, May 13. Available online: https://www.theguardian.com/world/2020/may/13/anti-asian-hate-crimes-up-21-in-uk-during-coronavirus-crisis (accessed on 30 November 2020).
Hamilton, Clive. 2018. *Silent Invasion: China's Influence in Australia*. Melbourne: Hardie Grant Books.
Harnisch, Sebastian, Sebastian Bersick, and Jörn-Carsten Gottwald. 2015. *China's International Roles: Challenging or Supporting International Order?* London: Routledge.
Hine, Christine. 2015. *Ethnography for the Internet: Embedded, Embodied and Everyday*. London and New York: Bloomsbury Academic, An Imprint of Bloomsbury Publishing PLC.
Hoffman, Aaron M. 2002. A Conceptualization of Trust in International Relations. *European Journal of International Relations* 8: 375–401. [CrossRef]
Human Rights Watch. 2020. Country Chapters: China's Global Threat to Human Rights. *World Report 2020*. Available online: https://www.hrw.org/world-report/2020/country-chapters/global (accessed on 24 July 2020).
Hvistendahl, Mara. 2020. *The Scientist and the Spy: A True Story of China, the FBI, and Industrial Espionage*. New York: Riverhead Books.
Jia, Xi. 2020. Chinese in the UK Donate $396,000 to Help Wuhan's Doctors Fighting Coronavirus. *CGTN*, Februaary 1. Available online: https://newseu.cgtn.com/news/2020-02-01/Chinese-in-the-UK-donate-396-000-to-help-Wuhan-s-doctors-NIcscNjxjG/index.html (accessed on 30 November 2020).

Kowalski, Bartosz. 2021. China's Mask Diplomacy in Europe: Seeking Foreign Gratitude and Domestic Stability. *Journal of Current Chinese Affairs* 50: 209–26. [CrossRef]

Kydd, Andrew. 2005. *Trust and Mistrust in International Relations*. Princeton: Princeton University Press. [CrossRef]

LCI. 2020. L'ambassade de Chine plaide le piratage après la publication d'un dessin polémique sur Twitter. *[Chinese Embassy Pleads Hacking after Controversial Cartoon Posted on Twitter*. May 25. Available online: https://www.lci.fr/international/tensions-etats-unis-chine-l-ambassade-chinoise-plaide-le-piratage-apres-la-publication-d-un-dessin-polemique-sur-twitter-2154696.html (accessed on 30 November 2020).

Le Monde. 2020. L'ambassadeur de Chine à Paris convoqué pour «certains propos» liés au coronavirus. [Chinese Ambassador to Paris Summoned for "Certain Remarks" Related to the Coronavirus]. February 15. Available online: https://www.lemonde.fr/sante/article/2020/04/15/l-ambassadeur-de-chine-a-paris-convoque-pour-certains-propos-lies-au-coronavirus_6036610_1651302.html (accessed on 30 November 2020).

Leach, William, and Paul Sabatier. 2005. To trust an adversary: Integrating rational and psychological models of collaborative policymaking. *American Political Science Review* 99: 491–503. [CrossRef]

Lieberthal, Kenneth, and Jisi Wang. 2012. Addressing U.S.-China Strategic Distrust. Available online: https://www.brookings.edu/wp-content/uploads/2016/06/0330_china_lieberthal.pdf (accessed on 23 July 2020).

Lipset, Seymour M., and Stein Rokkan, eds. 1967. Cleavage Structures, Party Systems, and Voter Alignments: An Introduction. In *Party Systems and Voter Alignments: Cross-National Perspectives*. New York: Free Press, pp. 1–64.

Lulu, Jichang. 2019. Repurposing Democracy: The European Parliament China Friendship Cluster. *Sinopsis*, November 26. Available online: https://sinopsis.cz/en/ep/ (accessed on 30 November 2020).

McGillivray, Fiona, and Alastair Smith. 2000. Trust and cooperation through agent-specific punishments. *International Organization* 54: 809–24. [CrossRef]

Mercer, David. 2020. Coronavirus: Hate Crimes against Chinese People Soar in UK during COVID-19 Crisis. Skynews. Available online: https://news.sky.com/story/coronavirus-hate-crimes-against-chinese-people-soar-in-uk-during-COVID-19-crisis-11979388 (accessed on 30 November 2020).

Murphy, Simon. 2020. Chinese People in UK Targeted with Abuse over Coronavirus. *The Guardian*. Available online: https://www.theguardian.com/world/2020/feb/18/chinese-people-uk-targeted-racist-abuse-over-coronavirus-southampton (accessed on 30 November 2020).

Oushinet. 2020. Yingguo huaqiao huaren qixin zhuli wuhan "kangyi" [Overseas Chinese in the UK Work Together to Help Wuhan in the "Fight against the Epidemic"]. Available online: http://www.oushinet.com/wap/qj/qjnews/20200202/340069.html (accessed on 30 November 2020).

Pak, Anton, Emma Mcbryde, and Oyelola A. Adegboye. 2021. Does High Public Trust Amplify Compliance with Stringent COVID-19 Government Health Guidelines? A Multi-country Analysis Using Data from 102, 627 Individuals. *Risk Management and Healthcare Policy* 1: 293–302. [CrossRef]

People's Daily. 2020. "Jiankang sichou zhilu" wei shengming huhang—kangji yiqing libukai mingyun gongtongti yishi [The "Health Silk Road" Escorts Life—The Fight against the Epidemic Is Inseparable from the Community of Common Destiny]. Available online: http://theory.people.com.cn/n1/2020/0324/c40531-31645276.html (accessed on 30 November 2020).

Phillips, Tom. 2017. EU Backs Away from Trade Statement in Blow to China's 'Modern Silk Road' Plan. *The Guardian*, May 15. Available online: https://www.theguardian.com/world/2017/may/15/eu-china-summit-bejing-xi-jinping-belt-and-road (accessed on 30 November 2020).

Qi, Jingwen, Stijn Joye, and Stijn Van Leuven. 2021. Framing China's mask diplomacy in Europe during the early covid-19 pandemic: Seeking and contesting legitimacy through foreign medical aid amidst soft power promotion. *Chinese Journal of Communication* 1–22. [CrossRef]

Rudolf, Moritz, and Stiftung Wissenschaft Und Politik. 2021. 'China's Health Diplomacy during Covid-19: The Belt and Road Initiative (BRI) in Action. *SWP Comment*. [CrossRef]

Ruzicka, Jan, and Nicholas Wheeler. 2010. The puzzle of trusting relationships in the Nuclear Non-Proliferation Treaty. *International Affairs* 86: 69–85. [CrossRef]

Saechang, Orachorn, Jianxing Yu, and Yong Li. 2021. Public Trust and Policy Compliance during the COVID-19 Pandemic: The Role of Professional Trust. *Healthcare* 9: 151. [CrossRef] [PubMed]

Seaman, John, and French Institute of International Relations (IFRI). 2020. COVID-19 and Europe-China Relations: A Country-Level Analysis. Available online: https://www.ifri.org/sites/default/files/atoms/files/etnc_special_report_covid-19_china_europe_2020.pdf (accessed on 25 March 2022).

Silver, Laura, Kat Devlin, and Christine Huang. 2020. *Unfavorable Views of China Reach Historic Highs in Many Countries—Majorities Say China Has Handled COVID-19 Outbreak Poorly*. Washington, DC: Pew Research Center. Available online: https://www.pewresearch.org/global/2020/10/06/unfavorable-views-of-china-reach-historic-highs-in-many-countries/ (accessed on 30 November 2020).

Silver, Laura, Kat Devlin, and Christine Huang. 2021. Large Majorities Say China Does Not Respect the Personal Freedoms of Its People. Pew Research Center. Available online: https://www.pewresearch.org/global/2021/06/30/large-majorities-say-china-does-not-respect-the-personal-freedoms-of-its-people/ (accessed on 1 December 2021).

Sohu. 2020. Yingguo henan tongxianghui qiaobao wei jiaxiang juanzeng kang"yi"wu [Overseas Chinese from the Henan Association of the United Kingdom Donated Anti-Epidemic Materials to Their Hometown]. Available online: https://www.sohu.com/a/371160088_160386 (accessed on 30 November 2020).

Statista. 2021. Level of Trust in Government in China from 2016 to 2021. Available online: https://www.statista.com/statistics/1116013/china-trust-in-government-2020/ (accessed on 10 January 2022).

Statista. 2022. Selected Countries with the Largest Number of Overseas Chinese 2020. Available online: https://www.statista.com/statistics/279530/countries-with-the-largest-number-of-overseas-chinese/ (accessed on 1 January 2022).

The State Council of the People's Republic of China. 2020a. Wang yi: Jianjue daying kangyi yiqing zujizhan tuidong goujian renlei mingyun gongtongti [Wang Yi: Resolutely win the Fight against the Epidemic and Promote the Building of a Community with Shared Future for Mankind]. Available online: http://www.gov.cn/guowuyuan/2020-03/01/content_5485253.htm (accessed on 30 November 2020).

The State Council of the People's Republic of China. 2020b. Zhonggong zhongyang zhengzhi ju changwu weiyuanhui zhaokai huiyi yanjiu jiaqiang xinxing guanzhuang bingdu ganran de feiyan yiqing fangkong gongzuo xijinping zhuchi huiyi [The Standing Committee of the Political Bureau of the CPC Central Committee Held a Meeting to Study and Strenghten the Prevention and Control of the Pneumonia Epidemic That Is Caused by the New Coronavirus Infection, the Meeting Was Chaired by Xi Jinping]. Available online: http://www.gov.cn/xinwen/2020-02/03/content_5474309.htm (accessed on 30 November 2020).

The White House. 2017. The National Security Strategy of the United States. December. Available online: https://www.whitehouse.gov/wp-content/uploads/2017/12/NSS-Final-12-18-2017-0905-2.pdf (accessed on 23 July 2020).

Thunø, Mette. 2018. China's New Global Position: Changing Policies towards the Chinese Diaspora in the 21st Century. In *China's Rise and the Chinese Overseas*, 1st ed. Edited by Bernard and Tan Chee-Beng Wong. London: Routledge, pp. 184–208.

Thunø, Mette. 2021. *Panel 9: Twitter Diplomacy*. Hong Kong Baptist University. YouTube. November 12. Available online: https://www.youtube.com/watch?v=fF7w_NXjybY (accessed on 1 January 2022).

Thunø, Mette. 2022. *Chinese Twitter*. Aarhus University Centre for Humanities Computing. Available online: https://github.com/centre-for-humanities-computing/chinese-twitter (accessed on 1 January 2022).

Tianjin Federation of Returned Overseas Chinese. 2020. Qing jiaxiang renmin shouxia women de xinyi!—Yingguo tianjin shanghui juanzeng wuzi qiyun [We Ask Our People to Receive Our Kind Regards—The UK-China Business Association Sends Out Donation Shipments]. Available online: http://www.tjql.org.cn/system/2020/02/09/020023050.shtml (accessed on 30 November 2020).

Torsten, Michel. 2016. 'Trust and International Relations'. *Oxford Bibliographies*. Available online: https://www.oxfordbibliographies.com/view/document/obo-9780199743292/obo-9780199743292-0192.xml (accessed on 23 July 2020).

Tran, Emilie, and Ya-Han Chuang. 2019. Social Relays of China's Power Projection? Overseas Chinese Collective Actions for Security in France. *International Migration* 58: 101–17. [CrossRef]

Tran, Emilie, and Yahia H. Zoubir. 2022. Introduction to the Special Issue China in the Mediterranean: An Arena of Strategic Competition? *Mediterranean Politics* 1–19. [CrossRef]

Tran, Emilie. 2022. Role dynamics and trust in France-China coopetition. *Mediterranean Politics*, 1–27. [CrossRef]

US Department of State. 2020. Communist China and the Free World's Future. In *Speech by Michael R. Pompeo, Secretary of State*. Available online: https://cl.usembassy.gov/secretary-michael-r-pompeo-remarks-communist-china-and-the-free-worlds-future/ (accessed on 1 January 2022).

Uslaner, Eric M. 2002. *The Moral Foundations of Trust*. Cambridge: Cambridge University Press.

Wang, Jisi. 2019. Assessing the radical transformation of U.S. policy toward China. *China International Strategy Review* 1: 195–204.

Wicks, Andrew C., Shawn L. Berman, and Thomas M. Jones. 1999. The Structure of Optimal Trust: Moral and Strategic Implications. *The Academy of Management Review* 24: 99. [CrossRef]

Xinhua. 2020a. Shandong fuying lianhe gongzuozu wancheng renwu huiguo [The Shandong Joint Working Group to Britain Completes Its Mission and Returns to China]. Available online: http://www.xinhuanet.com/politics/2020-04/03/c_1125811960.htm (accessed on 30 November 2020).

Xinhua. 2020b. Xi Says China's Battle against COVID-19 Making Visible Progress. Available online: http://www.xinhuanet.com/english/2020-02/19/c_138797580.htm (accessed on 30 November 2020).

Xinhua. 2020c. Xinhua Headlines: China Returns Solidarity with Europe in COVID-19 Battle. Available online: http://www.xinhuanet.com/english/2020-03/20/c_138898996.htm (accessed on 30 November 2020).

Zhao, Huanxin. 2020. US Sending Experts to Fight Virus. *China Daily*, January 30. Available online: https://global.chinadaily.com.cn/a/202001/30/WS5e324e46a310128217273b07.html (accessed on 30 November 2020).

Zhao, Lijian. 2020. 2020 nian 4 yue 10 ri wai jiao bu fa yan ren zhao li jian zhu chi li xing ji zhe hui [Foreign Ministry Spokesperson Zhao Lijian's Regular Press Conference on 10 April 2020—Embassy of the People's Republic of China in the Kingdom of Belgium]. Available online: http://be.chineseembassy.org/chn/fyrth/t1768268.htm (accessed on 30 November 2020).

Zhao, Suisheng. 2022. The US–China Rivalry in the Emerging Bipolar World: Hostility, Alignment, and Power Balance. *Journal of Contemporary China* 31: 169–85. [CrossRef]

Zoubir, Yahia H., and Emilie Tran. 2021. China's Health Silk Road in the Middle East and North Africa Amidst COVID-19 and a Contested World Order. *Journal of Contemporary China* 1–16. [CrossRef]

MDPI
St. Alban-Anlage 66
4052 Basel
Switzerland
Tel. +41 61 683 77 34
Fax +41 61 302 89 18
www.mdpi.com

Journal of Risk and Financial Management Editorial Office
E-mail: jrfm@mdpi.com
www.mdpi.com/journal/jrfm

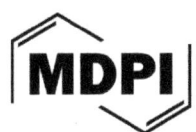

www.ingramcontent.com/pod-product-compliance
Lightning Source LLC
LaVergne TN
LVHW070558100526
838202LV00012B/498